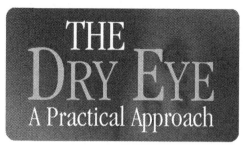

THE DRY EYE
A Practical Approach

For Butterworth Heinemann:

Publishing Director: Caroline Makepeace
Project Development Manager: Kim Benson
Project Manager: Derek Robertson
Design direction: George Ajayi

THE
DRY EYE
A Practical Approach

Sudi Patel BSc(Hons) MPhil PhD FCOptom FAAO
Optometric Adviser to the Common Services Agency, NHS Scotland, Edinburgh, UK
Visiting Professor, Institute of Ophthalmology, University
Miguel Hernandez de Elche, Alicante, Spain

Kenny J Blades BSc(Hons) PhD CBiol MIBiol
Clinical testing at an International Pharmaceutical Company, UK
Formerly Department of Optometry, Glasgow Caledonian University, Glasgow, UK

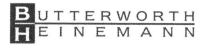

BUTTERWORTH
HEINEMANN

EDINBURGH LONDON NEW YORK OXFORD PHILADELPHIA ST LOUIS SYDNEY TORONTO

BUTTERWORTH-HEINEMANN
An imprint of Elsevier Science Limited

First published 2003

ISBN 07506 4978X

British Library Cataloguing in Publication Data
A catalogue record for this book is available from the British Library

Library of Congress Cataloging in Publication Data
A catalog record for this book is available from the Library of Congress

Note
Medical knowledge is constantly changing. As new information becomes available, changes in treatment, procedures, equipment and the use of drugs become necessary. The authors and the publishers have taken care to ensure that the information given in this text is accurate and up to date. However, readers are strongly advised to confirm that the information, especially with regard to drug usage, complies with the latest legislation and standards of practice.

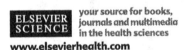

ELSEVIER SCIENCE
your source for books, journals and multimedia in the health sciences
www.elsevierhealth.com

The
publisher's
policy is to use
paper manufactured
from sustainable forests

Transferred to digital printing 2006
Printed and Bound by CPI Antony Rowe, Eastbourne.

Contents

Preface

The purpose of this book is to help you to understand, identify and manage dry eye, as it regularly presents to the optometrist. The authors have been presenting further education workshops on tear film evaluation and therapeutics together since 1994, and have become totally convinced of two things:

- the 'high street' optometrist is very interested in 'dry eye' because this condition presents frequently. Dry eye has been described as the single main problem likely to prevent a successful new contact lens fit. Furthermore, dry eye is a frequently encountered problem after ocular surgery involving the cornea.
- there is a need for a *simple* book to accompany the workshops we have been presenting: a text that can be read quickly and will clearly present the basic elements of tear film assessment and treatment.

It is the authors' intention to address these requirements, by presenting this book as a 'workshop in print'. In the following pages you will find answers to the commonest questions we have been asked over the years.

SP, KB 2003

Dry eye ready reckoner

Use this flow chart to help in your decision-making process

Before you assess your dry eye patient remember to:
- Focus on the relevant questions you should ask
- Decide on the clinical tests you should use

Use your findings to decide which treatments and procedures are best suited to your patient

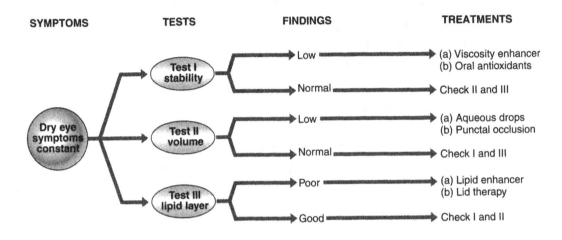

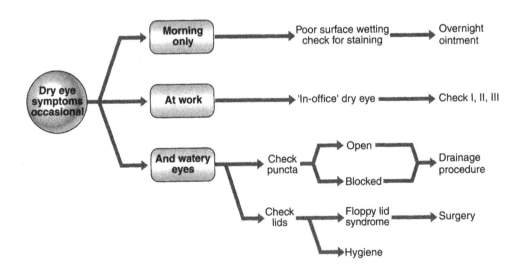

1 Introduction

By the end of this chapter you will understand:

■ The source, role and composition of the normal tear film;

■ What is meant by the term 'dry eye';

■ The different forms of dry eye encountered.

'Dry eye' is a generic term for a group of conditions characterized symptomatically by irritated, gritty, burning eyes, and clinically by alterations in the tear film and anterior surface of the eye. In a classic review, this syndrome was defined as 'a disorder of the tear film due to tear deficiency or excess tear evaporation which causes damage to the interpalpebral ocular surface and is associated with symptoms of ocular discomfort' (Lemp, 1995). This general definition encompasses a range of dry eye states with a range of etiologies.

Deficiencies in the production, quality or replenishment of the precorneal tear film will result in dry eye conditions. Such conditions can result in ocular surface damage, and may lead to eventual corneal damage and, ultimately, a detriment to visual performance.

Before considering the dry eye, it is important that we familiarize ourselves with the normal tear film and the underlying anatomy.

ROLES OF THE TEAR FILM

The tear film is a fluid that covers the cornea (the precorneal tear film) and the conjunctiva (the preocular tear film). It has been stated that the primary role of the tear film is to establish a refractive surface of high quality for the cornea and to ensure the well-being of the corneal and conjunctival epithelium. The roles of the pre-corneal tear film have been summarized as:

1. to protect the cornea from drying;
2. to maintain the refractive power of the cornea;
3. to defend against eye infection;
4. to allow gas to move between the air and the avascular cornea;
5. to support corneal dehydration (assisted by the tear film hyperosmolality).

As well as nurturing the cornea, the preocular tear film is necessary to protect the other epithelial tissues of the anterior surface (the bulbar and palpebral conjunctiva) from physical damage on blinking.

Under normal conditions, the tear film is of sufficient quantity and quality to fulfill the requirements outlined above.

Volume is an important issue: without a sufficient volume of tear fluid, a film cannot adequately form over the ocular surface and offer protection from exposure between blinks. An adequate volume of tears is also required if the tear film is to provide lubrication and prevent the shear forces of blinking from damaging the anterior eye.

Another important aspect is the tear film stability. The stability of the tear film is the property that allows it to maintain a confluent coverage of the ocular surface, for an adequate duration of time to protect the ocular surface between blinks. The tear film must also be of a sufficient quality, inherent of an adequate composition, to accomplish its numerous roles in the biophysical and bacteriostatic/bacteriocidal defense of the anterior surface.

STRUCTURE OF THE TEAR FILM

Several models describing the dimensions and layers of this complex film have been presented by dacryologists,[1] but the one presented by Holly and Lemp (1971, 1977) has been the most influential. The schematic representation of this model is found in Figure 1.1. This model describes a three-layered tear film that has an intrinsic relationship with the superficial epithelial layers of the

---

[1] Dacryologist: A person engaged in the study of tears and treatment of abnormal tear function.

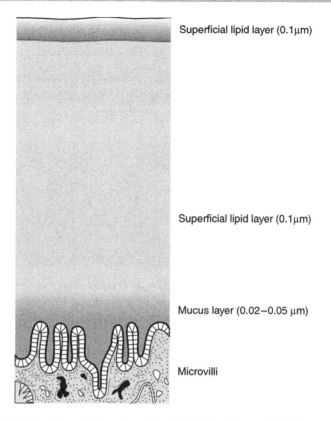

Superficial lipid layer (0.1μm)

Superficial lipid layer (0.1μm)

Mucus layer (0.02–0.05 μm)

Microvilli

Figure 1.1 Holly & Lemp's 3 Layer Tear Film Model (Holly & Lemp, 1977). From air to the microvilli present at the corneal epithelium.

cornea and conjunctiva. The innermost layer of the tear film is composed of a mucus layer, overlying which there is an aqueous phase. Above this is a layer of lipid.

Tiffany (1988) has proposed a slightly more complex model of the tear film, describing six layers (see Figure 1.2), the oily layer, the polar lipid monolayer, the adsorbed mucoid layer, the aqueous layer, the mucoid layer and the glycocalyx. The glycocalyx interfaces with the corneal/conjunctival epithelium, while the oily layer interfaces with air. This model takes into account additional layers and zones of interface not described by Holly and Lemp's model. It has been suggested that the mucus and aqueous 'layers' of the tear film should be considered simply as phases with more and less mucus respectively (Dilly, 1994).

The tear film has an estimated thickness of around 4–6 μm, being thickest immediately after the blink and subsequently thinning to a minimum of around 4 μm. These figures have been challenged, but are generally still accepted. Thinning occurs because the tear film is a dynamic structure under the influence of factors

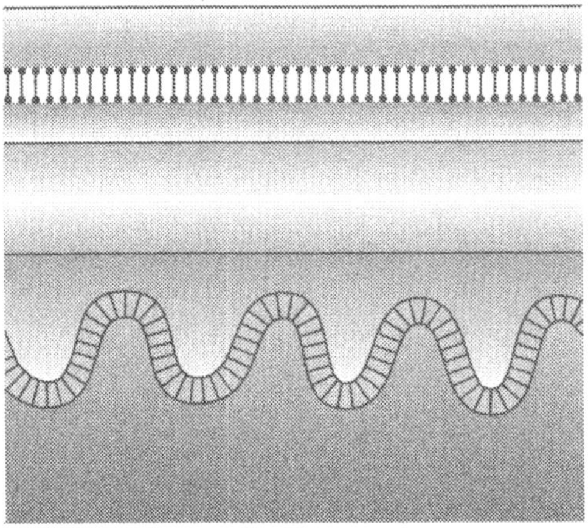

Air

Oily layer

Polar lipid monolayer

Adsorbed mucoid

Aqueous layer

Mucoid layer

Glycocalyx

Corneal epithelium

Figure 1.2 Tiffany's Model of the Tear Film (Tiffany, 1988). From air to the glycocalyx covering the microvilli of the corneal epithelium.

such as evaporation. Eventually the tear film ruptures and is reconstituted with each blink.

TEAR FILM COMPOSITION

Table 1.1 is a simple summary of the components and functions of the three main tear film layers. While the classic three-layered tear film model may not be completely accurate, or sufficient to explain the complex interactions between the phases of the tear film, it is useful to 'compartmentalize' the tear film into three layers when considering source and function of this complex structure, as it is how most of us were (and still are) taught at university.

A wide range of vitamins (e.g. A, C, E) and trace elements with anti-oxidant properties feature prominently in the various biochemical pathways leading to tear production. The essential 'ingredients' processed by the secretory apparatus to create the tear film are derived from the vascular system. An adequate diet, efficient absorption at the gut wall and reasonable conduction at the blood–tear secretory organ barrier are essential to maintain a healthy tear output.

The lipid layer

Even though we cannot be certain that there exists separate aqueous and mucus phases of the tear film, the lipid is certainly a

Table 1.1 Summary of the tear film

Layer	Source	Primary constituents	Primary roles
Lipid	Meibomian glands Glands of Zeis Glands of Moll	Cholesterol Fatty acids Fat	Prevents overflow Prevents skin lipid contamination Controls evaporation

Aqueous	Lacrimal glands
	Accessory lacrimal
	  glands (Krause &
	  Wolfring)
	Conjunctival
	  epithelium
	Corneal epithelium
		Water
		Inorganic electrolytes
		Organic substances
		  of low and high
		  molecular weights
			Gas exchange
			Antibacterial function
			Cleansing
			Optical surface
			  enhancement
			Lubrication

Mucus	Goblet cells
	Glands of Henle
	Glands of Manz
	Secretory epithelial
	  cells
		High carbohydrate to
		  protein ratio, cross
		  linked polymers
			Wetting and optical
			  surface enhancement
			  of epithelial tissue
			Physical/immunological
			  protection
			Cleansing

discrete layer. This layer is thought to be around 0.1 μm in thickness, and is spread over the ocular surface (and drags the aqueous phase along), by the sweep of the eyelids during each blink (Berger & Corrsin, 1974).

Source and composition of ocular lipid

The bulk of the lipid content of the tears is produced by the Meibomian glands, that open onto the eyelid margins. The lipid layer of the tear film contains a complex mixture of hydrocarbons, sterol esters, wax esters, triacylglycerol, free cholesterol, free fatty acids and polar lipids.

General roles of the lipid layer

The tear lipids deter overflow of the tear fluid, prevent wetting of the skin adjacent to the eye, and also allow for additional ocular lubrication. The tear lipid layer also plays a crucial role in the control of evaporation from the ocular surface (Craig & Tomlinson, 1997).

Decreased quality or quantity of the tear film surface lipid, as seen in Meibomian gland dysfunction, promotes the signs and symptoms of dry eye conditions. However, Craig and Tomlinson have shown that the tear evaporation rate only begins to increase when the lipid layer is breached, as even a thin but confluent lipid barrier can maintain control of evaporation. When the lipid layer is thickened, by manually expressing lipid from the Meibomian glands, tear film stability increases.

The aqueous layer

The aqueous phase of the tears is regarded by the traditional tear film models to be, by proportion, the greatest tear component, accounting for around 98% of the total thickness of the tear film. In the human tear film, this layer is believed to be around 7 μm thick.

Source and composition of the tear film aqueous phase

The majority of the aqueous phase is produced by the main and accessory lacrimal glands with additional water and electrolytes being secreted by the epithelial cells of the ocular surface. At least the main lacrimal gland secretion is under neuronal control, indicating minute-to-minute fine-tuning of the tear production rate, to match the requirement of fluid at the ocular surface.

The aqueous phase is a complex fluid composed primarily of water, with many solutes, including dissolved mucins, electrolytes and proteins. The comprehensive composition of the aqueous portion of the tear film reflects the diverse biochemical, biophysical and bacteriostatic functionality of this fluid (compare this with the equally complex composition and functionality of blood serum, for example).

The osmotic pressure associated with the tear film is primarily influenced by the relative concentrations of sodium, potassium and chloride ions present. The tear film's osmotic pressure is important in the control of cornea–tear film water flux. Bicarbonate and carbonate ions are important in pH buffering, maintaining the tear film pH at 7.3–7.6 when the eyes are open, as opposed to around 6.8 when the eyes are closed. (The tear film undergoes changes in the closed eye state, and takes some time to return to a 'normal' open eye state on waking. A discussion of the closed eye tear film is beyond the scope of this text, but may prove to be of interest, as extended wear contact lens use becomes more common.)

A high number of different proteins are also present, including immunoglobulins, albumins, lysozyme, lactoferrin, transferrin, histamine and glycoproteins. These are involved in, among other things, defense of the ocular surface against invading pathogens, and maintenance of tear film stability.

Tear proteins are markedly affected in the dry eye states, and this is the basis of one commercially available dry eye test, the Lactoplate™ test. (This test is discussed in Chapter 6.)

General roles of the aqueous phase

In addition to playing an optical role, the aqueous phase has several important functions. These include:

i) to provide an adequate lubrication between the moving surfaces of the eye and its adenexa;
ii) to remove foreign material;
iii) to nurture the corneal and conjunctival epithelia by keeping them in a moist state;
iv) providing nutrients needed by the epithelium;
v) allowing access to elements of blood for wound healing and bacteriostatic protection (Holly & Lemp, 1977).

Due to differences in viscosity between the aqueous and mucus phases of tears, the shear produced on blinking decreases rapidly within the mucus phase, reducing the shear forces affecting the epithelia to negligible levels. Without the lubrication provided by an adequate aqueous phase, the shearing forces produced on blinking would be transmitted directly to the epithelia through the mucus layer (Dilly, 1994), causing accumulative ocular surface damage.

The mucus layer

This layer is found sandwiched between the ocular surface and aqueous phase.

Sources and composition of ocular mucus

Ocular mucus is composed mainly of mucins in gel form, in complex with water, lipids, enzymes, other proteins, carbohydrates and electrolytes. The principal sources of ocular mucin are the goblet cells of the conjunctiva (which constitute the primary source), the glands of Manz in the limbal ring and the crypts of Henlé. Non-goblet cell secretory mucus vesicles constitute a secondary source of ocular surface mucins, and are responsible for construction of the glycocalyx. The glycocalyx gives a high-quality interface between the mucus layer and the epithelial cell surfaces, while separating the delicate ocular surface from the area of mucus where sheer occurs on blinking.

The theoretical requirements of mucus to allow wetting of the epithelial surface are debatable, however, the mucus layer *is* present in the healthy tear film, anchored at the epithelial microvilli and glycocalyx, and may be essential in overcoming temporary areas of non-wetting (as produced by desquamation or due to surface damage).

Under normal conditions, the mucus secreted by the conjunctival goblet cells is spread over the surface of the eye by the action of blinking. This forms a fine meshwork blanket of mucus which is only lightly adhered to the underlying glycocalyx, but more firmly attached at the outer surfaces of the goblet cells. This blanket of mucus forms a hydrophilic basement for the tear film. Debris and lipid (migrating from the superficial layer of the tear film tends to pollute the mucus), render some areas hydrophobic. The action of blinking rolls the contaminated, hydrophobic mucus into a fine mesh which then collapses to form the mucus strand found in the lower fornix. Simultaneously, the blinking action spreads fresh mucus from the goblet cells over the ocular surface, and so maintains a continuous hydrophilic interfacial surface.

General roles of the mucus layer

Viscosity of the tear fluid may be a major determinant of the tear film stability, and the major components likely to confer adequate viscosity are the tear proteins and mucous glycoproteins. Some ocular mucus becomes dissolved in the aqueous phase of the tear film, and this may also contribute to the stability of the film.

An adequate mucus layer is also required to physically protect the corneal and conjunctival epithelial cells from the assault of blinking and contact lens wear, and to fulfill its role as an immunoglobulin reservoir. Due to its micellar structure, this layer probably acts as an effective immunoglobulin reservoir, allowing their slow release over the day, when the open eye state renders the ocular surface more vulnerable to airborne pathogens.

The mucus layer quickly spreads to heal gaps and imperfections. The surface of the mucus layer is the first solid barrier encountered by invading material such as bacteria, therefore the rapid self repair of mucus layer imperfections is essential in protecting the epithelium against both localized surface drying effects and bacterial infiltration.

DRY EYE SYNDROMES

Dry eye has previously been reported as being of several classifications (Holly & Lemp, 1977).

Aqueous deficient dry eye

This is a partial or absolute deficiency of the aqueous phase of the tear film, and is a condition of fluctuating severity, most commonly developing in adults (especially post-menopausal females). Decreased aqueous production and decreased tear drainage can compromise the anterior surface, leading to an association between aqueous deficiency and secondary infections such as bacterial conjunctivitis and keratitis.

Mucus (soluble surfactant) deficiency

Decreased quantity or quality of surface mucus may lead to impaired surface wetting of the epithelia, and decreased lipid trapping and masking at the epithelial interface. Mucus deficiency is, like other forms of dry eye, associated with decreased tear stability. The majority of ocular mucus is produced by the conjunctival goblet cells, whose numbers are reduced by vitamin A deficiency (which promotes epithelial keratinization) and other tear deficiencies which compromise the ocular surface.

Lipid abnormalities

While complete tear film lipid deficiency is not known in man, alterations in lipid composition (as seen in chronic blepharitis) can decrease lipid function. This can cause decreased tear evaporation control and thus decrease tear film stability.

Lid surface abnormalities

When normal lid movement (blinking) is compromised, the area of cornea and conjunctiva not adequately served shows non-wetting. This poor wetting can lead to subsequent epithelial desquamation. Loss of tonus or paresis of one or more eyelid muscles may cause abnormal blinking.

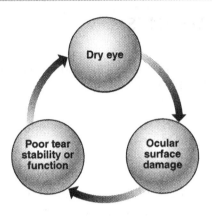

Figure 1.3 Dry eye: a cyclic disorder.

Epitheliopathy

The normal microvillous surface of the cornea is required to anchor the tear film (through interaction with the mucus phase). Any pathology adversely effecting the integrity of this epithelial surface decreases the tear film integrity, and thus stability, as demonstrated in Figure 1.3.

Lemp (1995) reported two major classes of dry eye:

1. Tear-deficient dry eye, where deficiencies of aqueous phase tear production or distribution lead to the most common form of dry eye.
2. Tear-sufficient (evaporative) dry eye, where sufficient tears are produced, but tear evaporation (due to a variety of factors) mediates dry eye signs and symptoms.

The *National Eye Institute/Industry Workshop on Clinical Trials in Dry Eyes* has provided a suggested dry eye classification scheme (Lemp, 1995). A summary of this is found in Figure 1.4. As can be seen from this classification scheme, evaporative dry eye encompasses mucus-deficient (surface changes), lipid-deficient and lid-related dry eye syndromes.

Thus, 'dry eye syndrome' is a term used to describe a variety of conditions, sharing common symptomatology and clinical signs, leading to a physical and functional breakdown of the tear film.

Such tear film disorders range in severity, from the borderline dry eye, which may only be apparent under conditions such as environmental challenge, to the severe (pathological) dry eye, as often found in Sjögren's syndrome.

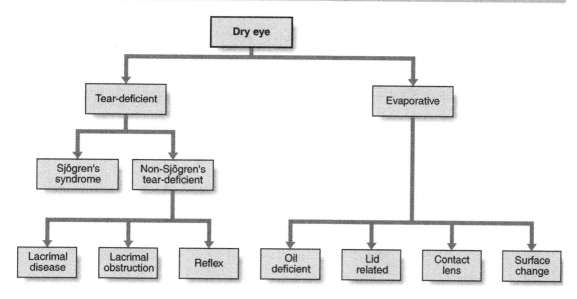

Figure 1.4 Dry eye classification after Lemp (1995).

REFERENCES

Berger R.E. and Corrsin S. (1974). A surface tension gradient mechanism for driving the pre-corneal tear film after blinking. *Biomechanics*, 7: 227–238.

Craig J.P. and Tomlinson A. (1997). Importance of the lipid layer in tear film stability and evaporation. *Optom Vis Sci*, 74: 8–13.

Dilly P.N. (1994). Structure and function of the tear film, In: *Lacrimal Gland, Tear Film And Dry Eye Syndromes: Basic Science And Clinical Relevance* (Sullivan D.A., ed.). Plenum Press, New York, pp 239–247.

Holly F.J. and Lemp M.A. (1971). Wettability and wetting of corneal epithelium. *Exp Eye Res*, 11: 239–250.

Holly F.J. and Lemp M.A. (1977). Tear physiology and dry eyes. *Surv Ophthalmol*, 22: 69–87.

Lemp M.A. (1995). Report of the National Eye Institute/Industry Workshop on clinical trials in dry eyes. *CLAO J*, 21: 221–232.

Tiffany J.M. (1988). Tear stability and contact lens wear. *J Br Contact Lens Assoc*, 11(s): 35–38.

2 Patient Self-Assessment

After this chapter you will have a better understanding of:

■ The sort of questions that you need to ask in order to determine if a dry eye is present;

■ How to rank the severity of symptoms;

■ How to numerically rate symptoms for monitoring purposes.

A clinician will examine bodily functions or organs depending on the presenting signs and symptoms. Unless there is a need for a health care check up, most people seek help after a bout of discomfort, pain or some other undesirable subjective phenomenon. Symptoms can fall into either subjective or objective categories. With the emphasis on preventative medicine over the last 50 years still to this day, many patients seek care for bodily functions when they experience subjective symptoms. The dry eye patient is no exception. Subjective symptoms range from mild occasional discomfort to severe constant pain. If the irritation is centered about the eye then how can we be sure it is related to dry eye? If the discomfort is not debilitating should the clinician still treat the dry eye? The short answer is yes. A hypothesis has been drawn linking ocular surface damage to lacrimal gland metabolism. Chronic long-term damage to the ocular surface does *not* trigger lacrimal activity to benefit the ocular surface. Instead, the response from the lacrimal gland could in the long run be more harmful than beneficial (Mathers, 2000). Thus, early intervention is indicated. By asking the patient to categorize the symptoms in a controlled manner it is possible to quantify the severity of the problem, monitor the condition and evaluate the effectivity of any subsequent therapy in a more clinically meaningful, less erroneous manner.

QUESTIONNAIRES

Patient assessment can be done in the waiting area by filling out a questionnaire administered by the clinical assistant or the patient him/herself. The responses may indicate ocular discomfort and the need for more specific clinical work-up. It would be useful to rate the severity of any discomfort using a numerical or alpha-numeric scale. Dry questionnaires range from the complex all-encompassing form featuring much detail (e.g. Lacrimedics questionnaire) to the simple questionnaire consisting of six basic questions (Bandeen-Roche *et al.*, 1997). The depth of discomfort can be recorded and appreciated at future check-ups by fellow clinicians. A long questionnaire is time consuming and the short one may miss out features relevant to the treatment modality. The McMonnies' questionnaire (McMonnies, 1986) is a well-balanced focused simple test that allows the patient to think about when the symptoms occur. If symptoms occur occasionally, the questionnaire allows us to pinpoint the source of provoked symptoms, e.g. do they present in certain environments. The McMonnies' questionnaire has been designed to determine:

- if the symptoms are constant or occasional; and
- if symptoms are related to external environmental factors or genuine intrinsic systemic factors.

The questionnaire not only informs the clinician but educates the patient. Questionnaires have been used to estimate the extent of dry eye in specific communities. Using the Bandeen–Roche system, the incidence of dry eye is probably 8% in people under 60, 15% in those between 60 and 80, 19% in those over 80 (Moss *et al.*, 2000). Begley *et al.* (2000) report about 50% of contact lens patients have dry eye problems whilst wearing their lenses. In a survey of office workers, using the McMonnies questionnaire 44% of respondents had dry eye symptoms either constantly and/or provoked by external factors such as cigarette smoke or air conditioning (Blades, 1997). Thus, when used as survey tools the results must be viewed with caution because, a survey depends on several factors such as:

  i) number and type (e.g. elderly, contact lens wearers, health) of subjects;
 ii) the genetic and general profile of the subjects;
iii) environment/location;
 iv) gender ratio;
  v) order and style of questions;
 vi) manner in which the questions were posed by the surveyor.

Within normals, tear stability and volume are reported to be higher in Caucasians compared with Chinese and Japanese subjects (Cho & Brown, 1993; Sakamoto *et al.*, 1993; Patel *et al.*, 1995). Factors such as these may have an impact on the incidence of dry eye in particular surveys. The questionnaire must be direct, unambiguous, take little time to fill out, be capable of yielding the information we require and be user-friendly. McMonnies' questionnaire has a simple scoring system based on the patient's answers, the higher the score the worse the condition. If a treatment is effective, at a later date the symptom score should reduce and this indicates numerically the subjective value of the treatment regimen. In terms of record keeping, symptom scoring replaces screeds of written notes with a single number. With treatment any changes in the score can be relayed back to the patient in a more meaningful, easy to comprehend manner. Thus resulting in better patient–practitioner communication and inter-relations.

VISUAL SCALES

Another, simpler, scoring system is the marked scale. For example a scale from say 'uncomfortable' to 'comfortable' in equal steps from 0 to 10 is a useful, visual, analog scale for scoring purposes. Analog scales are frequently used to estimate the extent and duration of systemic pain (Price *et al.*, 1983). They have been shown to be very useful for monitoring pain control after refractive surgery (Verma & Marshall, 1996). The advantages of such a scale are:

i) it is fast and easy to administer;
ii) the change in the score reflects the effectivity of a treatment plan;
iii) before and after scores can be recorded on the patient's record for future reference;
iv) the scale also allows the patient to monitor his or her own reaction/response to a treatment plan and allows the patient to more effectively compare different treatments.

The limitations of this kind of information must not be ignored. The disadvantages are:

i) As the patient is kept aware of his/her original symptom score, it could influence the subject score after treatment is administered.

ii) The score is non-parametric, hence standard parametric statistical tests cannot be used when assessing the usefulness of any treatment.

iii) Self-assessment questionnaires and scoring systems are not interchangeable.

For example in Figure 2.1, we have an analog scale showing results before and after treatment for a broad range of dry eye patients. On first glance, Figure 2.1 suggests the symptoms of the eight patients reduce after treatment, hence the treatments are beneficial. The scored data are *subjective*, so the results must be viewed with caution. In a clinical trial incorporating a placebo and using either trained or untrained subjects, the value of an analog scale can be strengthened by preventing subjects from seeing their previous scores. However, safe-guards like these cannot be easily incorporated into a busy clinical facility especially when the patient is asked to score symptoms in the place where the dry eye problems prevail (e.g. workplace or home). The result, or score, is true for that particular test scale but not for any other. Subjective scoring systems are intrinsically unique and their limitations must not be overlooked.

EXAMPLES OF DRY EYE QUESTIONNAIRES

Bandeen-Roche et *al.*, 1997

1. Do your eyes ever feel dry?
2. Do you ever feel a gritty or sandy sensation in your eye?
3. Do your eyes ever have a burning sensation?
4. Are your eyes ever red?
5. Do you notice much crusting on your lashes?
6. Do your eyes ever get stuck shut in the morning?

Allowable responses: never, rarely, sometimes, often or all the time.

Begley et *al.*, 2000

1. Do your eyes feel dry?
2. Do your eyes become sore?
3. Do your eyes feel scratchy or irritated?
4. Are your eyes sensitive to light?
5. Is your vision blurry or changeable?

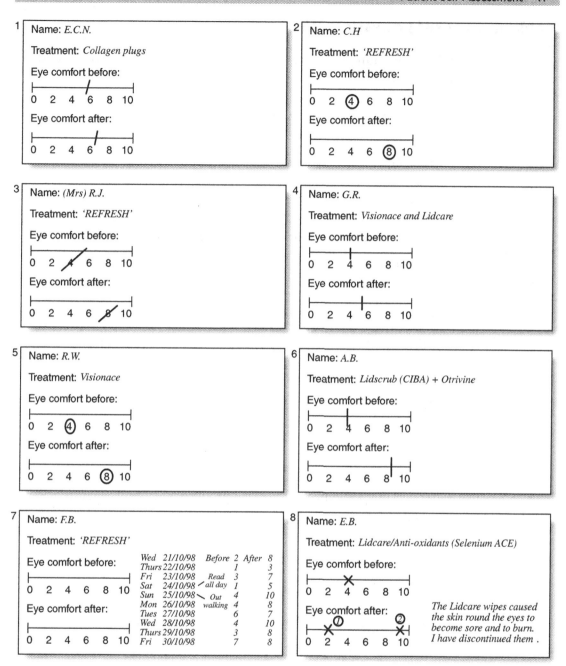

Figure 2.1 Patient identifiers have been removed. These are results from 8 separate patients with a variety of specific symptoms and treatments (e.g. drops, lid scrubs, punctal plugs).

Analog scale example:

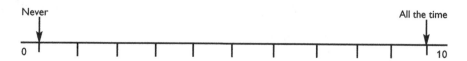

McMonnies (1986) questionnaire

N.B. The figures in parentheses are score values to individual responses.

1. Have you ever had drops prescribed or other treatment for dry eyes?

   Yes (2)
   No (1)
   Uncertain (0)

2. Do you ever experience any of the following symptoms?

   Soreness (1)
   Scratchiness (1)
   Dryness (1)
   Grittiness (1)
   Burning (1)

3. How often do you have these symptoms?

   Never (0)
   Sometimes (1)
   Often (2)
   Constantly (3)

4. Are you unusually sensitive to cigarette smoke, smog, air conditioning or central heating?

   Yes (2)
   No (0)
   Sometimes (1)

5. Do your eyes easily become very red and irritated when swimming?

   Not applicable (0)
   Yes (2)
   No (0)
   Sometimes (1)

6. Are your eyes dry and irritated after drinking alcohol?

   Not applicable (0)
   Yes (2)

No (0)
Sometimes (1)

7. Do you take

Antihistamine tablets or eye drops (1)
Diuretics [fluid tablets] (1)
Sleeping pills (1)
Tranquilizers (1)
Oral contraceptives (1)
Medication for digestive problems or duodenal ulcer (1)
Medication for high blood pressure (1)
Antidepressants (1)

8. Do you suffer from arthritis?

Yes (2)
No (0)
Uncertain (1)

9. Do you experience dryness of the mucous membranes such as the nose, mouth, throat, chest or vagina?

Never (0)
Sometimes (1)
Often (2)
Constantly (3)

10. Do you suffer from thyroid abnormality?

Yes (2)
No (0)
Uncertain (1)

11. Are you known to sleep with your eyes partly open?

Yes (2)
No (0)
Sometimes (1)

12. Do you have eye irritation as you wake from sleep?

Yes (2)
No (0)
Sometimes (1)

Lacrimedics

This is a record introduced by Lacrimedics Inc, Eastsound, WA, USA.

SYMPTOMS CHECKLIST

Print Name (Last) _____ (First) _____ Date: _____

Address: _____ Age: _____

_____ Sex M/F _____

Daytime Phone: (_____) Occupation: _____

What brings you to our office today? _____

CHECK THE SYMPTOMS YOU EXPERIENCE

	Left Eye	Right Eye	How Long		
Redness				Sinus congestion	
Dry eye feeling				Congestion	
Mucus or discharge				Post-nasal drip	
Sandy or gritty feeling				Cough–chronic	
Itching				Bronchitis chronic	
Burning				Head allergy symptoms	
Foreign body sensation				Seasonal allergies	
Constant tearing				Hay fever symptoms	
Occasional tearing				Cold symptoms	
Watery eyes				Middle ear congestion	
Light sensitivity					
Eye pain or soreness				Dry throat, mouth	
Chronic infection of eye or lid					
Sties, chalazion				Asthma symptoms	
Fluctuating visual acuity				Arthritis	
'Tired' eyes				Joint pain	
Contact lens discomfort					
Contact lens solution sensitivity					
Additional comments					
	YES				
Do you use lubricating eye drops?			What name brand?		
Do you wear contact lens?			How long have you had them?		
Are they comfortable?			Have you tried to wear them before and quit? Yes/No		

Do you wear glasses?		How long have you had them?
Have you ever had an eye injury?		Please describe:
Have you ever had eye surgery?		Please describe:
Are you allergic to anything?		Please list:
Do you take any medications?		List name and reason:

Are your eyes overly sensitive to (please circle): heaters, blowers, air conditioning, cigarette smoke, smog, pressurized airplane cabins, dust, pollen, video display terminal, sunshine, wind, contact lens wear?

Have you or a blood relative ever had: glaucoma, tuberculosis, lupus, gout, high blood pressure, cataracts, arthritis, diabetes, rheumatoid, thyroid disorder, heart disease, Sjögren's syndrome?

Patient's signature: _____

Doctor's signature: _____

REFERENCES

Bandeen-Roche K., Munoz B., Tielsch J.M. *et al.* (1997). Self reported assessment of dry eye in a population-based setting. *Invest Ophthal Vis Sci*, **38**: 2469–2475.

Begley C.G., Caffery B., Nichols K.K. *et al.* (2000). Responses of contact lens wearers to a dry eye survey. *Optom Vis Sci*, **77**: 40–46.

Blades K. (1997). *Investigation of the marginal dry eye and oral antioxidants.* PhD thesis, Glasgow Caledonian University.

Cho P. and Brown B. (1993). Review of the TBUT and a closer look at the TBUT of Hong Kong Chinese. *Optom Vis Sci*, **70**: 30–38.

Mathers W.D. (2000). Why the eye becomes dry: A cornea and lacrimal gland feedback model. *CLAOJ*, **26**: 159–165.

McMonnies C.W. (1986). Key questions in a dry eye history. *J Am Optom Assoc*, **57**: 512–517.

Moss S.E., Klein R. and Klein B.E. (2000). Prevalence of and risk factors for dry eye syndrome. *Arch Ophthalmol*, **118**: 1264–1268.

Patel S., Virhia S.K. and Farrell P. (1995). Stability of the precorneal tear film in Chinese, African, Indian and Caucasian eyes. *Optom Vis Sci*, **72**: 911–915.

Price D.D., McGrath P.A., Rafi A. and Buckingham B. (1983). The validation of visual analogue scales as ratio measures for chronic and experimental pain. *Pain*, **17**: 45–56.

Sakamoto R., Bennett E., Henry V.A. *et al.* (1993). The phenol red thread tear test – A cross cultural study. *Invest Ophthal Vis Sci*, **34**: 3510–3514.

Verma S. and Marshall J. (1996) Control of pain after photorefractive keratectomy. *J Refractive Surg*, **12**: 358–364.

3 Laboratory and Clinical Tests – A Balance

By the end of this chapter you will understand:

■ The difference between laboratory and clinical tests;

■ What to look for in a good clinical test, and what to avoid;

■ And appreciate the limits of your chosen tests.

LABORATORY VERSUS CLINICAL

The requirements of a good clinical test are very different to those of a good laboratory test. It is very important to keep this firmly in mind, given the great research interest in tears and the anterior eye. Many new techniques have been developed or adapted from other fields of science and technology, and applied to dacryology. The focus of this book is clinical, and the purpose of this chapter is to show that not all tests are of clinical relevance, even though they may be of great academic interest or have a unique research utility. Likewise, very simple tests may be of great use clinically, though out of favor in research labs.

Points to remember when considering whether to invest the time and resources required to add a new test or technique to your clinical 'arsenal' are the remit and resources of the task at hand. That is: what is the objective and how much time and money can be spent meeting this objective? A scientific research project may have a very narrow objective (say, to define the influence of a new contact lens material on a single tear parameter) and might be relatively well. In this situation, it would be very reasonable to spend a lot of time and money acquiring and mastering a new device or technique, even if it is only capable of showing a small average change in a single tear parameter across a large group of patients.

Let us contrast this with the needs of the main street eye care professional. In reality, assessment of the tears is only one of the remits addressed by a routine eye examination, even in contact lens practice, so will be resourced appropriately, in terms of time (to master and perform on each occasion) and money (to purchase, maintain and routinely use). Also, a test must be capable of indicating the status and highlighting untoward changes in an *individual* patient, to be of clinical utility.

Is there a cut-off value? – What does it mean?

Ideally, a clinical test should have a cut-off value or grading scheme. For example, a Schirmer test result of under 10 mm in 5 minutes is indicative of borderline dry eye (test inadequacies not withstanding – see Chapter 5 for a discussion of this topic). Likewise, a non-invasive tear thinning time of under 10 seconds is indicative of borderline dry eye. These tests have established, diagnostic cut-off values (10 mm and 10 seconds) that can be used to classify *individual* patients (with varying degrees of success from patient to patient – though beyond the scope of this text, many statistical texts handle the concepts of clinical test sensitivity and specificity in detail). Without recognized, adopted cut-off values, it is often difficult to apply clinical tests on an individual patient basis. Often a new test shows promise, but may not be truly, widely useful until there is enough collective clinical experience to adopt an agreed diagnostic cut-off value or clinical grading scheme. The repeatability of a given test and the appropriateness of the diagnostic cut-off value or grading scheme used often defines a technique's value in clinical practice. Even without a diagnostic cut-off value, a sound test may be useful for tracking an individual patient's response to treatment or disease progression, so the lack of a diagnostic cut-off value does not mean a test is not useful – common sense must be applied on a test-by-test basis.

Unfortunately, there is no single predictive test for dry eye, in either the clinical or the scientific arena.

Most dacryologists would suggest that the clinician is best advised to employ a selection of simple tests to assess *tear film stability, tear volume, ocular surface health and symptoms*, and to apply these systematically.

Finally, it is a cliché, but the only useful test is one that is used. If a 'lab on a chip' device was developed that could accurately measure, say, tear protein profiles, it would undoubtedly offer great potential for the routine diagnosis and follow up of dry eye patients. However, if a single-use device cost as much as the price of a typical eye examination, it would be very unlikely to find its way into common main street clinical practice, in the UK at least. It should, however be remembered that most new clinical tests started in a lab somewhere.

FEATURES OF CLINICAL TESTS AND TECHNIQUES

- Able to indicate tear/ocular surface problems in individuals (perhaps in concert with other tests).
- Preferably has an accepted diagnostic cut-off value or grading scheme.
- Should be as simple, inexpensive and quick to perform as possible.
- The more commonly available the better.

Examples of clinical tests*

- Tear Break Up Time (TBUT) – Despite being inferior to non-invasive alternatives, this is a widely available test, requiring only a slit lamp and a drop of fluorescein. A result of under 10 seconds is considered low.
- Non-Invasive Break Up Time (NIBUT) – widely available, as can be performed using a Tearscope or Tearscope plus. A result of under 10 seconds is considered low.
- Tear Thinning Time (TTT) – very widely available as can be performed using the mires of a Bausch & Lomb keratometer. A result of under 10 seconds is considered low.
- The Schirmer test – the ubiquitous test of tear production. A result of less than 10 mm wetting in 2 minutes is considered low.
- Tear Meniscus Height – a rapid non-invasive test of tear volume gaining much popularity.
- Hyperemia assessment – there are several widely available charts.
- Corneal and conjunctival staining – using Rose Bengal – (this should probably be reserved for severe dry eye) or fluorescein.
- Slit lamp examination – though not really a 'test' this is integral to screening for dry eye problems.

---

* In the Authors' opinions – others may differ in their opinions regarding the classification of these tests and techniques.

FEATURES OF LABORATORY TESTS AND TECHNIQUES

- Able to identify minute changes in tear/ocular surface parameters with high resolution.
- Can be considered useful even if the results are only meaningful across relatively large samples of patients.
- Can be complicated, expensive and/or time consuming.

Examples of laboratory tests[*]

- High Performance Liquid Chromatography (HPLC) – can be used to assess tear fluid composition. This is costly, time consuming and technically demanding.
- Clifton nanoliter Osmometry – this measures how salty the tears are. Time consuming and technically demanding, but probably the *gold standard* test for dry eye.
- Impression cytology and flow cytology – a way of assessing the status of the ocular surface. Attempts have been made to use cytological methods as a clinical tool, but this is too time consuming and demanding for routine clinical utility.
- Evaporimetry – to assess how well the lipid layer of the tears retards evaporation – this requires expensive equipment and is too time consuming for routine clinical use.

Examples of tests that are questionably clinically orientated[*]

- The Phenol Red Thread Test (PRT) – designed to be a quick and less irritating alternative to the Schirmer test, this test has yet to prove itself in the 'real world'. It is still not clear exactly what this test is measuring, or what diagnostic cut-off value should be adopted.
- Automated Osmometry – recent attempts to automate the assessment of tear osmolality must be applauded, but have not yet put this test within the reaches of main street practitioners. The authors hope that these attempts will be continued, as routine tear osmolality assessment would be of great clinical utility if the technique could be made quick, simple and inexpensive enough.

Further information on the tests and procedures mentioned in this section are referenced in subsequent chapters.

4 Stability of the Tear Film

By the end of this chapter you will understand:

■ The concepts of tear stability and tear break up;

■ Methods that are used to assess tear stability;

■ How to improve your tear stability assessment in clinical practice.

TEAR FILM STABILITY AND BREAK UP

An important factor, when considering the quality of the tears and ability of this fluid to function for the protection and maintenance of the anterior ocular surface, is the stability of the precorneal and preocular tear films.

The tear film is reformed by the actions of the eyelids upon blinking, approximately every 3–6 seconds. If the eye is kept open following a blink, the tear film can be seen to rupture, exposing dry spots of uncovered epithelium. In many dry eyes, the tear film ruptures before the blink, exposing the epithelium; or the blink rate is greatly increased to try to prevent this from happening. The ability of the tear film to maintain its form between blinks is of paramount importance, however the mechanisms of tear film rupture and, in fact, the underlying principles governing the tear film stability are not fully understood.

Formation of the tear film has been explained in terms of surface tensions and solid surface free energies. The drop in free energy on eye closure is believed to favor wetting of the ocular surface, allowing the tear film to form. As the eyelids open, following the blink, the tear film is dragged into place. Initially, the eyelid pulls the lipid with it as the eye opens, then the lipid drags the aqueous layer upwards from the meniscus.

Once formed, the property that maintains tear film integrity is described as tear film stability. The tear film is a delicate and dynamic structure, and its stability is probably a consequence of a variety of factors. The stability of this film has been attributed to the influences of several factors:

- adequate lipid layer coverage;
- an adequate mucus phase;
- sufficient quality of the epithelial surfaces of the cornea and conjunctiva;
- aqueous phase viscosity.

It seems likely that a harmonious interaction between all of these factors is essential for *optimal* tear film stability.

The tear film is transient. After a finite period of time the integrity of the tear's structure is lost, leading to tear film rupture (and, thus, loss of confluent coverage of the ocular surface). We do not know exactly why or how the tear film ruptures, but two major theories have been advanced.

Holly and Lemp (1977) have suggested that migrating lipids contaminate small areas of the mucus phase of the tear film. This

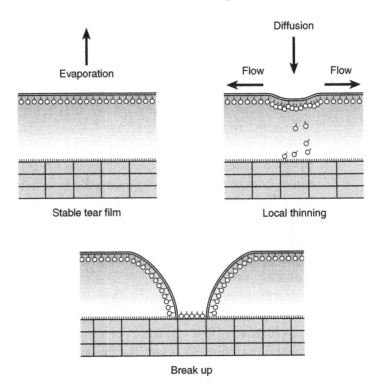

Figure 4.1 Holly & Lemp's model of tear film break up. Contaminating lipids cause decreased epithelial wettability, leading to tear film break up (Holly, 1980).

makes areas of the mucus phase hydrophobic and, so, unable to support the aqueous phase of the tear film. This model is depicted in Figure 4.1.

An alternative and more complicated model (Sharma & Ruckenstein, 1985; Ruckenstein & Sharma, 1986) has also been proposed. It is argued that the mucus phase is susceptible to the influences of short-range intermolecular interactions. A 'two-step, double film' mechanism of tear rupture has been proposed (this model is depicted in Figure 4.2).

1. Immediately following tear film reformation (by the blink), the thinner areas of the mucus layer at the tips of the epithelial cell microvilli begin to thin under the influence of interaction forces. Simultaneously, the aqueous phase begins to thin, due to evaporation and drainage. As mucus phase deformation continues, the mucus layer ruptures and retards to form mucus islands. This allows the aqueous layer to come into direct contact with the epithelial surface.

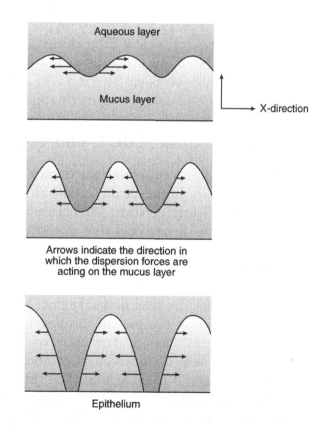

Figure 4.2 Sharma & Ruckenstein's model of tear film break up. Local dispersion forces within the thin mucus layer cause mucus layer rupture. This renders the exposed areas of epithelium unable to support a stable tear film (Ruckenstein & Sharma, 1986).

2. The relatively hydrophobic epithelial surface is unable to support the aqueous phase of the tear film. For this reason, the tear film subsequently ruptures, exposing small areas of naked epithelium.

Although the exact mechanism underlying tear film stability and, inevitably, break up is not known, the measurement of break up time (as an indication of the tear film stability) is a unique parameter. As such it provides useful information regarding the tear film, and cannot be replaced by other methods of investigation.

TESTS OF TEAR STABILITY

Many tests have been devised to investigate the ability of the tear film to adequately cover the otherwise exposed anterior surface of the eye, for a sufficient duration of time to prevent drying and subsequent damage to the underlying tissues. The tear film is respread and reformed every few seconds on the blink, and tear film stability is taken to be insufficient if break up occurs in under 10 seconds.

Tear film stability assessment techniques can be considered as invasive or non-invasive. This is a very important distinction, as the non-invasive techniques are greatly superior to the invasive method.

Invasive tear break up time (TBUT, fluorescein break up time)

This test requires observing the cornea using a slit lamp biomicroscope, with a broad-beam cobalt-blue light source set at, say, 10× magnification (Norn, 1969; Lemp & Hamill, 1973). To view the tear film, fluorescein dye is instilled, e.g. by wetting a dry fluorescein-impregnated paper strip (e.g. Fluoret™ by Smith and Nephew) with a drop of saline and placing on the bulbar cornea for a brief moment. The dye readily mixes in the tear fluid and after 1 or 2 blinks the tear film takes on a uniform fluorescent green appearance. Ask the patient to refrain from blinking and in most cases within 60 seconds dark spots or streaks will form within the tear film. These discontinuities in fluorescence indicate breaks in the continuity of the tear film. The time elapsing between a complete blink, and the appearance of the first 'dark spot or streak' is measured and taken to be the 'break up time'. Five successive measures are routinely taken, and the mean value calculated. In dry eyes break up time is usually less than 10 seconds.

Several workers have suggested this invasive break up time assessment to be of poor repeatability and questionable validity, probably due to:

i) The destabilizing effect of fluorescein on the tear film itself.
ii) The volume of fluorescein added is uncontrolled and relatively large compared with the natural tear reservoir.
iii) Contact with the ocular surface will initiate some reflex lacrimation.

For these reasons, many workers have turned to the non-invasive tear film stability assessment techniques (see below).

However, we live in the real world and many people *do* still perform TBUT as their standard assessment of tear stability. If you do not have access to a non-invasive method of assessing tear stability, then it is far better to perform TBUT than to not assess tear film stability at all. The usefulness of the TBUT test can be increased by minimizing the amount of fluorescein used. This has two clear advantages:

1. this prevents 'quenching' of fluorescence;
2. this minimizes the destabilizing effects of the fluorescein, so should give more valid assessment results.

A much smaller amount of fluorescein can be instilled using a new proprietary fluorescein-impregnated paper strip with a tapered tip (the Dry Eye Test or DET™, Ocular Research Boston, Boston, USA). If these are not available, then you could trim regular fluorets to a narrow tip using sterile scissors (disposable scissors can be bought from laboratory suppliers if you have no means of sterilizing metal scissors).

Non-invasive tests of tear film stability

Non-invasive assessment of tear stability was first mooted in the 1980s. The first device for non-invasive measurement of tear film stability was presented by Mengher *et al.* (1985). This consisted of a large hemispherical bowl featuring thin white illuminated parallel criss-cross lines on a dark background. The subject is seated, the bowl is arranged to reflect the lines off the cornea and the reflection is observed using a microscope. Other techniques based on the same optical principles are the keratometer mire (Patel *et al.*, 1985),

HIRCAL grid (Hirji *et al.*, 1989), Loveridge grid (Loveridge, 1993) and a portable device constructed from a wok (Cho, 1993). The instrument devised by Mengher *et al.* is bulky and this limits its appeal in routine clinical practice.

The fundamental principles common to these techniques are based on the reflective properties of the smooth, stable tear film. As the tear film distorts (as it thins), its ability to reflect, undistorted, a regular optical array or pattern diminishes. The time elapsing between a complete blink, and the appearance of the first distortion is measured and taken to be the 'tear thinning time' (TTT). Five successive measures are routinely taken, and the mean value calculated. In essence, non-invasive tests of tear stability are based on observing the quality and stability of the first Purkinje image.

The HIRCAL grid (Hirji *et al.*, 1989) comprises a Bausch and Lomb Keratometer, modified by removing one of the doubling prisms and including a white grid etched on a black plate, in place of the original mires. The grid is projected onto the surface of the tears. Breakdown of the tear film as observed with the HIRCAL grid is shown in Figure 4.3. One possible disadvantage of this technique concerns the limited area of precorneal tear film which may be examined using the HIRCAL grid (approximately the central zone of 3 mm in diameter). It is conceivable that an artificially high TTT may be recorded, due to the delay between the occurrence of peripheral localized tear thinning, and the observation of this thinning as it spreads to the viewable central area.

The Loveridge grid is, essentially, a miniaturized, hand-held HIRCAL grid (Loveridge, 1993), and as such appears to offer less magnification and a poorer image quality than the HIRCAL grid, though it does cover a larger overall area of the cornea.

The Bausch and Lomb Keratometer can also be used to measure TTT, using the standard mires as a light pattern source (Patel *et al.*, 1985). However, the mires cover a smaller total area of the cornea, and so may be more difficult to accurately use than the HIRCAL grid, leading to an artificial delay between tear thinning and its observation.

Corneal topographers based on the Placido disc can also be used to assess tear stability. The video monitor in most computerized photokeratoscopes is used to align the instrument and record the Purkinje images when crisp and sharp. By asking the patient to blink and observe the time taken for part of the reflected image to breakdown in clarity you can measure tear stability and widen the potential of the videokeratoscope. Ancillary staff trained to operate the videokeratoscope could also assess tear stability.

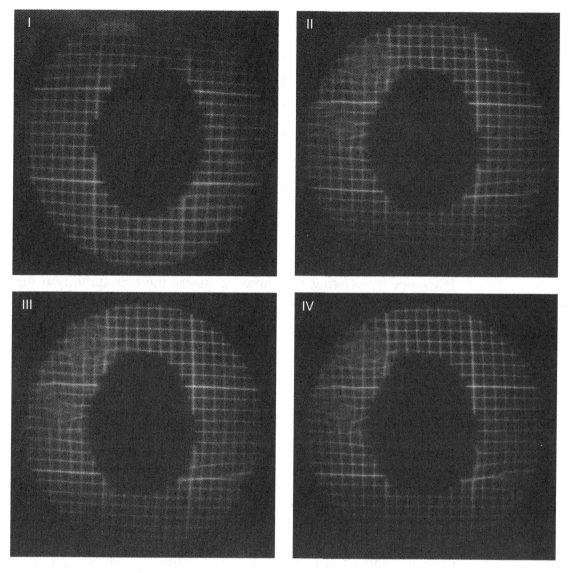

Figure 4.3 Breakdown of the precorneal tear film observed using HIRCAL grid. I: pre-rupture.
II to IV: change in appearance as tear film continues to breakdown at 10 and 4 o'clock.

A device not reliant on the first Purkinje image is the Keeler Tearscope™, an instrument which provides a wide field, specularly reflected view of the anterior surface, using a diffuse hemispheric light source. This light source is a cold cathode, which used in conjunction with a non-illuminated slit-lamp biomicroscope provides a semi-quantifiable assessment of lipid layer thickness. By measuring the time between a blink and the appearance of the first discontinuity in the lipid layer, the non-invasive break up time (NIBUT) can be measured (Guillon & Guillon, 1994). The Keeler

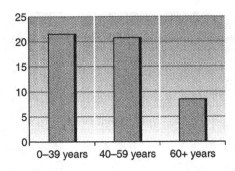

Figure 4.4 Tear thinning time and age. Stability in seconds. Subject age grouping shown on X axis (0–39, $n = 52$, S.D. $= \pm12.7$ seconds. 40–59, $n = 27$, S.D. $= \pm17.5$ seconds. 60+, $n = 31$, S.D. $= \pm6.9$ seconds. Patel *et al.*, 2000).

Tearscope Plus™ that superseded the original Tearscope was supplied with a flexible grid insert. This expanded the use of the Tearscope by offering the choice to assess the tear stability using the first Purkinje image and/or lipid layer by specular reflection.

The various non-invasive tear film stability assessment techniques can be considered in terms of those which measure the tear thinning time (TTT), and those which measure the non-invasive break up time (NIBUT). NIBUT is believed to be a measure of the time taken for a discontinuity in the superficial lipid layer of the tear film to occur following a blink, whereas TTT is a measure of the time taken for the tear film to thin, following a blink. Tear thinning is believed to occur just prior to tear break up. For this reason, TTT and NIBUT are taken to be similar parameters, not interchangeable or synonymous, but both indicative of tear film stability. In real life use, however, there is far less difference between the NIBUT and TTT than between either of these parameters and TBUT, and so the distinction between tests of NIBUT and TTT are probably only of academic relevance. Before introducing any tear stability measurement into your clinical routine you should practise the technique and develop your own age-matched 'norms'. The stability of the tear film reduces with age. Judged by measuring TTT, this effect is most noticeable after the age of 60 years, as shown in Figure 4.4.

A crucial but frequently overlooked advantage of any non-invasive test is its value in assessing the tear film over either rigid or soft contact lenses, *in situ*.

Improved assessment success and comfort

Patients are often unable to refrain from blinking for a sufficient period of time to allow tear stability to be assessed. It is often found that this is the case in patients with a relatively high tear stability when a non-invasive method of assessment is used (as patients are not used to refraining from blinking for over 30 seconds).

There are a number of strategies that can be adopted to deal with this problem. Each has its own benefits and drawbacks.

1. **Train the patients to refrain from blinking.** Patients do get better at refraining from blinking with a little practice. This will give a good measurement of tear stability, but takes too long for routine clinical work.
2. **Truncate the data.** Is there really any clinical advantage in knowing that your patient has a tear stability of over, say, 45 seconds? If a patient's tear film is still stable at 45 seconds, then record the stability as '<45 seconds' and let the patient blink. This reduces the quality of data, so it would not be suitable for clinical research, but is fine for clinical practice.
3. **Anesthetize the patient.** A single drop of benoxinate hydrochloride 0.4% in each eye 5 minutes before assessing the tear film will help the patient to refrain from blinking. This has been shown to have no effect on mean tear stability (Blades *et al.*, 1999). Unfortunately, this does sting a little, and tear stability cannot be assessed for 5 minutes after the anesthetic is instilled. This has limited practical appeal except in those cases where the clinician wants assurance that there is no reflex component affecting tear stability.

SUMMARY

To serve the anterior ocular surface, the tears must be of adequate stability, so it is important to routinely assess tear film stability. A variety of tear stability tests are available. These can be categorized as invasive or non-invasive tear stability assessment techniques. It is widely agreed that non-invasive tests of tear stability are preferred.

REFERENCES

Blades K.J., Murphy P.J. and Patel S. (1999). Tear thinning time and topical anesthesia as assessed using the HIRCAL grid and the NCCA. *Optom Vis Sci*, 76: 164–169.

Cho P. (1993). Reliability of a portable non-invasive tear break-up time test on Hong Kong-Chinese. *Optom Vis Sci*, 70: 1049–1054.

Guillon J.P. and Guillon M. (1988). Tear film examination of the contact lens patient. *Contax* **May 14–18**: 14–18.

Guillon J.P. and Guillon M. (1994). The role of tears in contact lens performance and its measurement. In: *Contact Lens Practice* (Guillon M. and Rubens M., eds). Chapman Hall Medical, London, p 462.

Hirji N., Patel S. and Callander M. (1989). Human tear film pre rupture time (TP-RPT): A non invasive technique for evaluating the pre corneal tear film using a novel keratometer mire. *Ophthal Physiol Opt*, **9**: 139–142.

Holly F.J. (1980). Tear film physiology. *Am J Optom Physiol Opt*, **57**: 252–257.

Holly F.J. and Lemp M.A. (1977). Tear physiology and dry eyes. *Surv Ophthalmol*, **22**: 69–87.

Lemp M.A. and Hamill J.R. (1973). Factors affecting tear film breakup in normal eyes. *Arch Ophthalmol*, **89**: 103–105.

Loveridge R. (1993). Breaking up is hard to do. *Optom Today*, **33**(21): 18–24.

Mengher L.S., Bron A.J., Tonge S.R. and Gilbert D.J. (1985). Effect of fluorescein instillation on the precorneal tear film stability. *Curr Eye Res*, **4**: 9–12.

Norn M.S. (1969). Dessication of the precorneal tear film. I: Corneal wetting-time. *Acta Ophthalmol*, **47**: 865–880.

Patel S., Murray D., McKenzie A., Shearer D.S. and McGrath B.D. (1985). Effects of fluorescein on tear break-up time and on tear thinning time. *Am J Optom Physiol Opt*, **62**: 188–190.

Patel S., Boyd K.E. and Burns J. (2000). Age, stability of the precorneal tear film and the refractive index of tears. *Contact Lens & Anterior Eye* **23**: 44–47.

Ruckenstein E. and Sharma A. (1986). A surface chemical explanation of tear film break up and its implications. In: *The Pre Ocular Tear Film In Health, Disease And Contact Lens Wear* (Holly F.J., ed.). Dry Eye Institute, Lubbock, Texas, pp 697–727.

Sharma A. and Ruckenstein E. (1985). Mechanism of tear film rupture and its implications for contact lens tolerance. *Am J Optom Physiol Opt*, **62**: 246–253.

5 Assessment of Tear Volume

By the end of this chapter you will understand:

■ The key features in the development of modern methods for assessing tear volume;

■ The limitations of the commonly used techniques;

■ How to incorporate simple non-invasive tests as part of your clinical routine.

Estimates for the volume of tears covering the ocular surface range from $2.74 \pm 2.0\,\mu L$ (Mathers *et al.*, 1996) to $7\,\mu L$ (Mishima *et al.*, 1966). The bulk of this volume is made up of fluid secreted by the main (primary) and secondary lacrimal glands. As you read this chapter tears are passively secreted and flowing onto your ocular surfaces and in a few seconds you will blink. This will force tear fluid towards the lacrimal puncta and, via these two anatomical landmarks the tears will pass from the ocular surface and into the lacrimal canaliculae. Intuitively, a dry eye is one with low tear volume. How can we measure tear volume in the clinical setting? Tests for tear volume are either invasive or non-invasive.

INVASIVE TESTS FOR TEAR VOLUME

Schirmer test

One of the earliest tests for estimating tear volume was devised by Schirmer (1903). This is a strip of thin filter paper (45 mm long, 5 mm wide) which is hooked over the lower eyelid. The hook is 5 mm long with a rounded edge. On contact with the ocular surface the paper absorbs tears. The length of paper wetted over a set time of 5 minutes is an indication of tear volume. The paper can irritate the ocular surface initiating a reflex action whereby the volume of tears secreted by the lacrimal glands increases. Thus, the Schirmer test is measuring both a basal and reflex tearing. By anesthetizing the ocular surface with say, 0.4% benoxinate or 0.5% amethocaine, it is claimed the reflex stimulation is prevented and a true measure of basal tear secretion can be made (Jones, 1966; Lamberts *et al.*, 1979; Jordan & Baum, 1980; Clinch *et al.*, 1983). The Schirmer strip comes into contact with not only the ocular surface but also the lid margin and some lashes. This suggests that, maybe the lid margins should also be anesthetized if the aim is to measure basal tear secretion. Many investigators conclude that the Schirmer test measures the flow of tears rather than volume and the fact that it irritates the ocular surface is a useful adjunct. If the Schirmer score is still low after irritating the ocular surface then clearly we have a very dry, as opposed to a marginally dry, eye. Low Schirmer test results are encountered when corneal sensitivity is reduced in severe dry eyes (Xu *et al.*, 1996). Furthermore, Schirmer test results are low after refractive surgery presumably because corneal sensitivity has been reduced (Ozdamar *et al.*, 1999; Aras *et al.*, 2000). The Schirmer test has been criticized for its poor reproducibility, it is time consuming, it is irritating and has poor diagnostic value especially when attempting to investigate the marginal dry eye (Feldman & Wood, 1979; Patel *et al.*, 1987; Cho & Yap, 1993a,b). A dry–normal cut-off value of 5 mm of wetting in 5 minutes has been used for many years but this is not reliable because 17% of normal eyes have a Schirmer wetting of less than 5 mm (Wright & Meger, 1962) and 32% of dry eyes have a Schirmer wetting of greater than 5 mm (Farrell *et al.*, 1992). The true value of the Schirmer test in the modern setting is questionable, even though it is still one of the most popular tests used by clinicians. Examples of typical reported values for the Schirmer test are shown in Figure 5.1.

Cotton thread test

Cotton can soak up tear fluid by capillary action. The cotton thread (Kurihashi, 1978; Hamano *et al.*, 1982) is dyed with a pH-sensitive phenol red which changes from yellow-orange to red-orange on contact with tears. This is useful for quickly checking the length of wetted thread. The volume of tears taken up by the thread depends on the exact type of cotton and the duration of insertion. The Hamano thread is inserted for 15 seconds and is

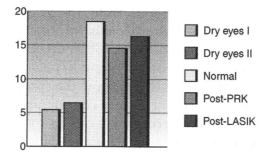

Figure 5.1 Some examples of Schirmer test results (mm). Dry Eyes I (Farrell *et al.*, 1992, n = 34, average age 56 years). Dry Eyes II (Xu *et al.*, 1996, n = 44, average age 52.5 years). Normals (Xu *et al.*, 1996, n = 26, average age 50.2 years). Post-PRK (Ozdamar *et al.*, 1999, n = 32). Post-LASIK (Aras *et al.*, 2000, n = 28).

marketed in several countries under the trade name Zone-Quick™ (Showa Inc., Japan). This thread is 70 mm long with a 3 mm hook at one end. The lower lid is gently depressed and the 3 mm hook is placed over the lower lid margin, on to the conjunctiva about half the distance from the center towards the outer canthus. The patient is asked to relax and keep looking straight ahead. Alternatively, the patient could just keep the eyes closed. After removing the Zone-Quick thread from the ocular surface the soaked up tears continue to flow along the thread. It is good practice to measure the length of wetting as soon as the thread is removed to reduce the effect of this systematic error. The soft thin cotton is less irritating compared with the relatively stiffer Schirmer paper strip and more likely to infer basal tear volume (Hamano *et al.*, 1982). This is not completely true because within normals the tear meniscus height (see later, Tear Meniscus Height) tends to increase during the 15 seconds of thread insertion (Blades *et al.*, 1999). Using the Zone-Quick thread, dry eyes tend to wet below 10 mm, averaging at 6.9 mm (Mainstone *et al.*, 1996). Wetting values for normal eyes range from 15.4 mm (Cho & Kwong, 1996) to 27.4 mm (Little & Bruce, 1994). It appears that within normals, differences in thread wetting values are related to ethnic variations. If you decide to use these threads you should establish baseline normal values for the patients within your community.

A custom-made phenol red cotton tear test can be produced easily using simple products (e.g the GCU thread described by Blades & Patel (1996)). The flow rate of tears along the thread depends on the duration of insertion quality, type and ply of the cotton. Instead of 15 seconds of insertion Cho and Yap (1994) recommended 60 seconds and for our thread we found 120 seconds was suitable based on flow dynamics. But, not all dry eyes are aqueous deficient. However, using the 0.2 mm diameter 50 mm long GCU thread for a cut-off value of 20 mm the sensitivity and specificity values were 86% and 83%, respectively, between aqueous-deficient and non-aqueous-deficient dry eyes (Patel *et al.*, 1998). The practical value of this is clear, if the clinician suspects a dry eye because of the type and variety of symptoms, the thread can quickly help decide if the problem is caused by an aqueous deficiency or otherwise. In turn, this helps the clinician decide what treatment regimen should be initiated. Does the thread measure tear flow or volume? A correlation between tear flow and thread wetting has not been substantiated (Tomlinson *et al.*, 2001). It could be that the tear fluid present at the ocular surface is absorbed when the thread is first inserted and, once this is depleted to a critical mass, reflex lacrimation is stimulated and the subsequent tears soaked up by the thread represents the tear flow at that point in time. Exactly what the thread measures at any moment during use is still open to question.

The population of post-operative cataract and treated glaucoma patients is predicted to rise substantially over the next decade, increasing the pool of potential dry eye patients. Cataract surgery involving the cornea can lead to dry eye symptoms. Adrenergic beta-blockers are used to treat glaucoma and can affect lacrimal protein secretion leading to changes in tear composition and dry eye symptoms (Mackie *et al.*, 1977; Coakes *et al.*, 1981). Typical GCU thread-wetting values for treated glaucoma and pseudophakic patients with dry eye symptoms are compared with other aqueous-deficient and non-aqueous-deficient dry eyes in Figure 5.2. Clearly, these two groups are analogous with the aqueous-deficient dry eyes and should be treated accordingly to combat discomfort.

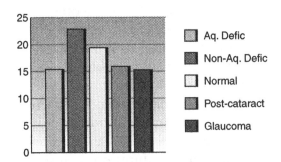

Figure 5.2 Typical wetting values (mm) for a custom Phenol Red Thread (GCUT). Aqueous deficient, (Patel *et al.*, 1998, n = 35, average age 53 years). Non-Aqueous deficient (Patel *et al.*, 1998, n = 24, average age 63 years). Normal (Blades and Patel, 1996, n = 20, average age 56 years). Post-cataract (n = 40, average age 75 years). Treated glaucoma (n = 36, average age 77 years).

Fluorophotometry

Fluorophotometry is a laboratory-based system used to measure tear flow and turnover rates. A controlled measure of fluorescein is instilled in the eye and the fluorescence is gauged over time. The rate of decay in fluorescence indicates tear flow and turnover. By extrapolation it is possible to predict the tear volume at the moment of fluorescein instillation. To be precise, the tear evaporation rate is required to make the final calculation. Fluorophotometric data indicate that the measurement of tears using the phenol red cotton test is not related to tear flow (Tomlinson *et al.*, 2001). It must be borne in mind that both tests are invasive and this in itself can affect the parameter under investigation.

NON-INVASIVE TESTS FOR TEAR VOLUME

Tear meniscus height and curvature

The tear meniscus is bound between the ocular surface, lid margin and the air. The surface exposed to the air is concave and cylindrical. The distance from the lid margin to the boundary between the ocular surface and the edge of the tear rivulus is the tear meniscus height (TMH). It is claimed that 75–90% of the total fluid covering the ocular surface is contained within the upper and lower tear menisci (Holly, 1986). The volume of fluid contained in the lower meniscus is the product of length and area of cross-section. In turn, the area of cross-section is dependent on the TMH and the curvature of the meniscus (TMC). It follows that the height and/or curvature of either the lower or upper tear meniscus is proportional to tear volume. In clinical practice TMH can be measured quickly and reliably at a magnification of 30× or more using a graduated eyepiece. The resolution can be improved by increasing the magnification, for example using a video capture system the magnification can be over 100×. Furthermore, measurement of TMH is a useful non-invasive technique for investigating not only the dry eye but also the patient complaining of occasional epiphora. If the TMH is consistently high there may be a partial blockage of the naso-lacrimal drainage system requiring treatment. Optical doubling devices are often included in either the eyepiece or objective of microscopes as an aid to mensuration because these items can improve both accuracy and repeatability when measuring relatively small dimensions (e.g. the optical pachometer for corneal thickness measurement). To this end, doubling devices have been used to measure TMH (Port & Asaria, 1990). This has not achieved mainstream popularity for the following reasons:

i) The technique is time consuming and there is a learning curve associated with its use.
ii) Keeping the eyes open beyond the normal inter-blink interval and the extended exposure to the bright light of the slit lamp tends to promote reflex lacrimation.
iii) The apparatus may not allow measurement away from the central horizontal region of the tear meniscus.

The busy clinician needs to measure ocular features quickly, with a reasonable level of both accuracy and repeatability. Slit-lamp video capture and eyepiece graticules satisfy the needs of the busy clinician. When the lid margin is irregular (e.g. in elderly patients or after injury), the TMH can be reliably assessed in a region where the margin is relatively regular. Using the slit lamp it can be difficult to decide where exactly the tear meniscus tapers off and ends. After some practice adjusting the incident and viewing beams of the slit lamp the clinician soon learns to identify the junction where the tear meniscus ends. An example of a TMH of 0.3 mm in an elderly patient is shown in Figure 5.3. This was measured using an eyepiece graticule and 32× magnification. Figure 5.4 shows the TMH over a soft lens to be much lower at 0.07 mm. The TMH over monthly replacement soft lenses is typically 40–50% less than the TMH normally encountered at the ocular surface without the lens (Figure 5.5). This strongly suggests that the tear fluid available to moisten the lens surface is not optimal.

The subjective measure of TMH is a relative, not an absolute, measurement because it depends on the observer's interpretation of where the base of the tear meniscus starts and where the top of the tear meniscus ends. Mainstone et al. (1996) instilled fluorescein as an aid to view the tear meniscus and reported mean TMH values of 0.46 mm (S.D. ± 0.17 mm) in normals and 0.24 mm (S.D. ± 0.09 mm) in dry eyes. Instillation could stimulate reflex lacrimation and, according to Oguz et al. (2000) TMH in dry eyes increased by 26% from 0.19 mm (S.D. ± 0.09 mm) to 0.24 mm (S.D. ± 0.11 mm) after introducing fluorescein, but the change was not significant. Statistical tests may not have detected a change but the clinical value of this difference cannot be ignored.

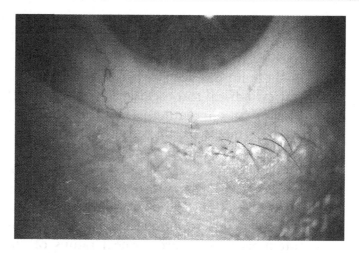

Figure 5.3 Tear meniscus height. Lower tear meniscus height (TMH) of 0.3 mm. This is the length of the perpendicular from the edge of the lower eyelid to the boundary between tear meniscus and ocular surface. Note, in this case an eyelash is trapped in a notch in the lower lid margin.

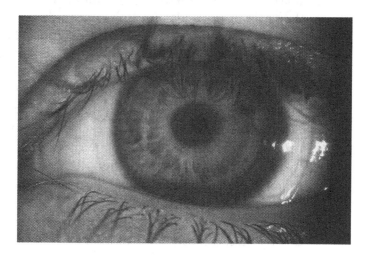

Figure 5.4 Tear meniscus over a soft contact lens. Lower tear meniscus height (TMH) of 0.07 mm. This is approximately 50% of the TMH normally encountered over the ocular surface.

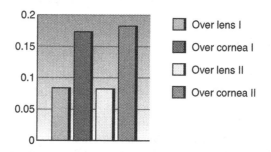

Figure 5.5 Typical values for tear meniscus height (TMH). I, lower TMH (mm) anterior to Focus™ (CibaVision) monthly replacement lenses and cornea ($n = 46$, difference statistically significant, $p < 0.0001$). II, lower TMH (mm) anterior to Surevue™ (Vistakon) monthly replacement lenses and cornea ($n = 28$, difference statistically significant, $p < 0.0001$).

TMC has been measured by recording a cross-section of the tear meniscus, photograbbing the image and later using curve-fitting techniques (Mainstone *et al.*, 1996). A non-invasive attachment for a slit lamp has been developed utilizing the reflective properties of the cylindrical tear meniscus (Yokoi *et al.*, 1999; Oguz *et al.*, 2000). A series of alternating parallel black and white lines is reflected off the tear meniscus, the size of the reflection is directly proportional to the TMC. Most authors quote values for tear meniscus curvature in units of mm. Strictly speaking these quotes are for *tear meniscus radius* (TMR). *Curvature* is defined as the reciprocal of radius therefore a TMR of 0.2 mm is equivalent to a true TMC of $5 \, mm^{-1}$. The errors in this technique are similar to the errors encountered in attempts to measure corneal radius of curvature. A keratometer could be modified to measure the radius of curvature of the tear meniscus. The resolution of keratometry is limited by diffraction theory to +/−0.04 mm (Charman, 1972). The average TMR is 0.37 mm in normals and 0.26 mm in dry eyes (Yokoi *et al.*, 2000a) hence the error in a single measurement of TMR could be 11% and 15%, respectively. TMR is highly correlated with TMH (Oguz *et al.*, 2000). Therefore, measuring TMH could be used to infer TMR if preferred. Using a video-capture technique to measure TMH, it can be shown that the tear volume does not remain constant with PRT insertion. We would expect the TMH to reduce as tears are soaked up by the thread. This is not the case, TMH increased significantly from 0.41 mm to 0.51 mm after 15 seconds of thread use, suggesting reflex lacrimation does occur during use of this thread in normals (Blades *et al.*, 1999). On the other hand, in dry eyes using a TMC (sic) method others have shown tear volume appears fairly constant during thread insertion (Yokoi *et al.*, 2000b).

Armed with a good slit lamp, an image recording system or eyepiece graticule, tear volume can be clinically assessed, non-invasively and reliably, on condition magnification is greater than 30×.

REFERENCES

Aras C., Odamar A., Bahcecioglu H., Karacorlu M., Sener B. and Ozkan S. (2000). Decreased tear secretion after laser in situ keratomileusis for high myopia. *J Refract Surg*, **16**: 362–364.

Blades K.J. and Patel S. (1996). The dynamics of tear flow within a phenol red impregnated thread. *Ophthal Physiol Opt*, **16**: 409–415.

Blades K.J., Patel S., Murphy P.J. and Pearce E.I. (1999). Is there a reflex component of phenol red thread wetting? *Optom Vis Sci*, **76**(suppl): 228.

Charman W.N. (1972). Diffraction and the precision of measurement of corneal and other small radii. *Am J Optom Arch Am Acad Optom*, **49**: 672–680.

Cho P. and Kwong Y.M. (1996). A pilot study of the comparative performance of two cotton thread tests for tear volume. *J Br Contact Lens Assoc*, **19**: 77–82.

Cho P. and Yap M. (1993a). Schirmer test I: A review. *Optom Vis Sci*, **70**: 152–156.

Cho P. and Yap M. (1993b). Schirmer test II: A clinical study of its repeatability. *Optom Vis Sci*, **70**: 157–159.

Cho P. and Yap M. (1994). The cotton thread test on Chinese eyes: effect of age and gender. *J Br Contact Lens Assoc*, **17**: 25–28.

Clinch T.E., Benedetto D.A., Felberg N.T. and Laibson P.R. (1983). Schirmer's test – A closer look. *Arch Ophthalmol*, **101**: 1383–1386.

Coakes R.L., Mackie I.A. and Seal D.V. (1981). Effects of long term treatment with timolol on lacrimal gland function. *Brit J Ophthalmol*, **65**: 603–605.

Farrell J., Grierson D.J., Patel S. and Sturrock R.D. (1992). A classification for dry eyes following comparison of tear thinning time with Schirmer tear test. *Acta Ophthalmol*, **70**: 357–360.

Feldman F. and Wood M.M. (1979). Evaluation of the Schirmer tear test. *Can J Ophthalmol*, **14**: 257–259.

Hamano H., Hori M., Mitsunaga S., Kojima S. and Maeshima J. (1982). Tear secretion test (a preliminary test). *Jap J Clin Ophthalmol*, **32**: 103–107.

Holly F.J. (1986). Tear film formation and rupture: an update. In: *The Preocular Tear Film in Health, Disease and Contact Lens Wear* (Holly F.J., ed.). pp 634–645. Dry Eye Inst, Lubbock, Tx.

Jones L.T. (1966). The lacrimal secretory system and its treatment. *Am J Ophthalmol*, **62**: 47–60.

Jordan A. and Baum J.L. (1980). Basic tear flow: Does it exist? *Ophthalmology*, **87**: 920–930.

Kurihashi K. (1978). Fine thread method and filter paper method of measuring lacrimation. *Jap J Clin Ophthalmol*, **28**: 1101–1107.

Lamberts D.W., Foster S. and Perry H.D. (1979). Schirmer test after topical anesthesia and tear meniscus height. *Arch Ophthalmol*, **97**: 1082–1085.

Little S.A. and Bruce A.S. (1994). Repeatability of the phenol-red thread and tear thinning time tests for tear function. *Clin Exp Optom*, **77**: 64–68.

Mackie I.A., Seal D.V. and Pescod J.M. (1977). Beta-adrenergic receptor blocking drugs: tear lysozyme and immunological screening for adverse reaction. *Brit J Ophthalmol*, **61**: 354–359.

Mainstone J.C., Bruce A.S. and Golding T.R. (1996). Tear meniscus measurement in the diagnosis of dry eye. *Curr Eye Res*, **15**: 653–661.

Mathers W.D., Lane J.A. and Zimmerman M.B. (1996). Tear film changes associated with normal aging. *Cornea*, **15**: 229–334.

Mishima S., Gasset A., Klyce S.D. and Baum J.L. (1966). Determination of tear volume and flow. *Invest Ophthalmol Vis Sci*, **5**: 264–276.

Oguz H., Yokoi N. and Kinoshita S. (2000). The height and radius of the tear meniscus and methods for examining these parameters. *Cornea*, **19**: 497–500.

Ozdamar A., Aras C., Karakas N., Sener B. and Karacorlu M. (1999). Changes in tear flow and tear stability after photorefractive keratectomy. *Cornea*, **18**: 437–439.

Patel S., Farrell J. and Bevan R. (1987). Reliability and variability of the Schirmer test. *Optician*, **194**(5122): 12–14.

Patel S., Farrell J., Blades K.J. and Grierson D.J. (1998). The value of a phenol red impregnated thread for differentiating between the aqueous and non-aqueous deficient dry eye. *Ophthal Physiol Opt*, **18**: 471–476.

Port M.J.A. and Asaria T.S. (1990). Assessment of human tear volume. *J Brit Contact Lens Assoc*, **13**: 76–82.

Schirmer O. (1903). Studies of the physiology and pathology of the secretion and drainage of tears. *Arch Ophthalmol*, **56**: 197–291.

Tomlinson A., Blades K.J. and Pearce E.I. (2001). What does the phenol red thread test actually measure? *Optom Vis Sci*, **78**: 142–146.

Wright J.C. and Meger G.E. (1962). A review of the Schirmer test for tear production. *Arch Ophthalmol*, **67**: 564–565.

Xu K.P., Yagi Y. and Tsubota K. (1996). Decrease in corneal sensitivity and change in tear function in dry eye. *Cornea*, **15**: 235–239.

Yokoi N., Bron A.J., Tiffany J.M., Brown N., Hsuan J. and Fowler C. (1999). Reflective meniscometry: a non-invasive method to measure tear meniscus curvature. *Br J Ophthalmol*, **83**: 92–97.

Yokoi N., Bron A.J., Tiffany J.M. and Kinoshita S. (2000a). Reflective meniscometry: a new field of dry eye assessment. *Cornea*, **19**(3 Suppl): 37–43.

Yokoi N., Kinoshita S., Bron A.J., Tiffany J.M., Sugita J. and Inatomi T. (2000b). Tear meniscus changes during cotton thread and Schirmer testing. *Invest Ophthalmol Vis Sci*, **41**: 3748–3753.

6 Assessment of Tear Quality

By the end of this chapter you will understand:

■ The key features in the development of modern methods for assessing tear quality;

■ The limitations of the commonly used techniques;

■ How to incorporate simple non-invasive tests as part of your clinical routine.

TEAR QUALITY IN GENERAL

The biochemical composition of the tear samples can be evaluated using a variety of lab-based tests. In this chapter we will concentrate on the clinical tests you can incorporate into your practice and routine with minimal intrusion.

SLIT LAMP

The slit lamp is the ideal tool to investigate:

i) ocular surface cellular damage using vital stains such as Lissamine Green, Rose Bengal or Fluorescein;
ii) debris contaminating the tears;
iii) meibomian openings and oil droplets at the lid margins;
iv) lashes for general state of hygiene, health and signs of inflammation;
v) contact lens, surface quality, movement and post-lens debris.

Contact lens-induced dry eye (CLIDE) can be associated with poor surface wetting, gradual build up of deposits, lens dehydration or accumulation of post lens debris. Changing the fit or cleaning regimen, use of wetting agents, altering wearing schedules, include occasional ocular washouts are techniques that are often used to combat CLIDE. The slit lamp will help you quickly decide what is the likely cause of CLIDE and what you should implement. Ideally, the patient should be examined after wearing the lenses for a few hours because symptoms of CLIDE tend to occur later in the day.

LID MARGIN, CANTHI AND STAINING

Meibomian gland dysfunction is commonly associated with skin conditions such as acne and psoriasis. Examples of waxy and oily meibomian secretions are shown in Figures 6.1 and 6.2.

On many occasions a patient's dry eye symptoms are related to poor hygiene and/or blocked meibomian gland openings. Tear foam (saponification) is a sign of changing tear biochemistry especially with regard to the lipids. Foam can be detected at the canthi mainly in the older patients as shown in Figure 6.3.

Fluorescein may be instilled to detect regions of erosion or poor wetting, an example is shown in Figure 6.4. Patients with dry eye symptoms on waking up may sleep with the eyes not fully closed. Such patients are easily detected with vital stains.

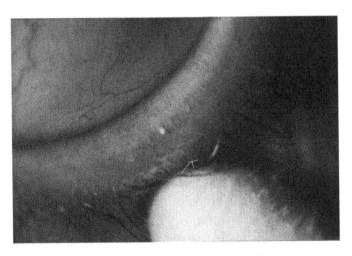

Figure 6.1 Waxy secretion from a meibomian gland. Gentle squeezing with fingers or using a cotton bud will express any wax.

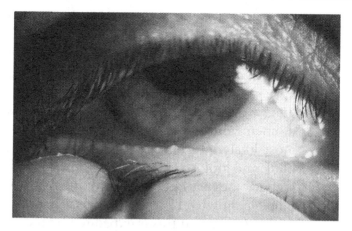

Figure 6.2 Oily secretion from a meibomian gland. Gentle squeezing with fingers or using a cotton bud will express any wax.

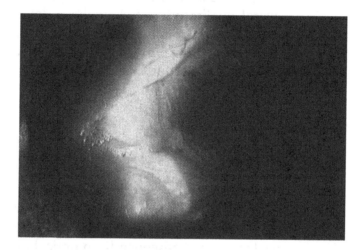

Figure 6.3 Tear saponification. Froth forming at the inner canthus.

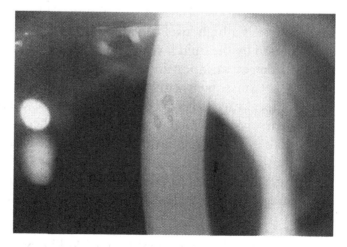

Figure 6.4 Fluorescein break up. Regions of poor wetting have either incomplete wetting or rapid local tear break up after the blink.

The slit lamp check is a relatively simple fast procedure, however it gives us little information regarding tear structure and no information on tear biochemistry. It would be wrong to equate tear debris with dry eyes simply because patients with dry eye symptoms can have relatively 'clean' tears. Many patients present with 'dirty' polluted tears and complain of no symptoms whatsoever. From the moment you started to read this paragraph you blinked at least once most likely you blinked 3 or 4 times. Why did you blink? If you blink and look straight ahead your eyes will feel fine but, after a few seconds they will become uncomfortable. Most people will need to blink again after 15 seconds. This is because the tear film has started to destabilize and this is expedited by the presence of debris. Where ocular surface sensitivity is depressed, the individual may not experience the discomfort, consequently there are no symptoms.

Several qualitative tests have been developed, here we will discuss the tests which have had a major impact on tear research and understanding, concentrating on those tests which could be easily incorporated into your clinical practice.

THE LIPID LAYER

The lipid layer is essential in reducing the rate of tear evaporation, the thicker the layer the lower the evaporation rate (Craig & Tomlinson, 1997). A stable, uniform thick layer is desirable. Lipid has a refractive index greater than the underlying aqueous component of the precorneal tear film, consequently an optical interference pattern can be generated by the lipid layer using an appropriate illuminating system (Doane, 1989; Guillon & Guillon, 1993; King-Smith et al., 1999). There is a high level of variability in the interferometric pattern generated by the lipid layer because optical interferometry has the power to detect variation in thickness within thin films to a resolution of $\lambda/2$. Consequently, the appearance can vary over the cornea because of local variations in lipid layer thickness. Keeler produced a portable Tearscope™ which could be used to check for contaminants such as make up and regularity of the tear menisci in addition to assessing the lipid layer. A picture chart is provided to assist in grading the interference pattern. Broadly speaking, the pattern can be categorized subjectively in increasing thickness as follows.

- Grade 1: No lipid.
- Grade 2: Marmoreal (a marble-like pattern either open or closed meshwork, up to 50 nm).

- Grade 3: waves, flow (50–80 nm).
- Grade 4: Amorphous, featureless pattern (80–90 nm).
- Grade 5: Color fringes (greater than 90 nm).

This non-invasive device is well suited for examining the tear film over contact lenses *in vivo*, a typical example is shown in Figure 6.5. In the majority of cases, the lipid layer in front of soft lenses is almost non-existent as noted in Figure 6.6. Glaucoma patients treated with beta-blockers and post-cataract patients often present with dry eye symptoms (see Chapter 5). In Figure 6.7, the distribution of lipid layer thickness in some patients is compared with age/gender matched normals. Clearly, the lipid layer tends to be thin in these three groups but there is no real inter-group difference. After refractive surgery such as LASIK, many complain of dry eye symptoms and for no obvious reason this group tends to present with a thinner lipid layer as noted in Figure 6.7.

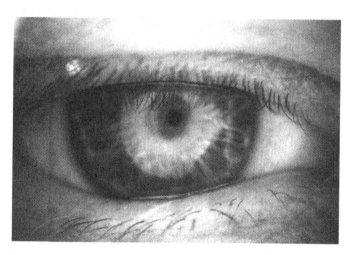

Figure 6.5 Thin lipid layer over a soft contact lens observed using the Tearscope™. The device also highlights the tear meniscus.

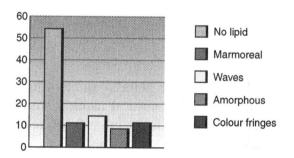

Figure 6.6 Percentage distribution of lipid layer types over a daily disposable soft lens (1-day Acuvue, *n* = 35).

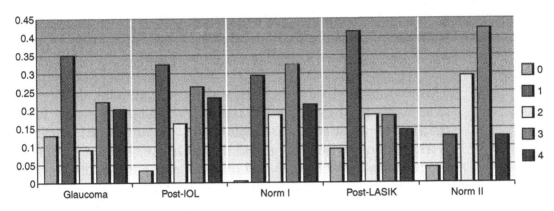

Figure 6.7 Distribution of tear lipid layer types in: Treated glaucoma (*n* = 46). Post-cataract surgery (*n* = 31), Post-LASIK (*n* = 22, Patel *et al.*, 2001). Norm I (*n* = 34) and Norm II (*n* = 24) are the appropriate age and gender matched normals. 0 = No lipid. 1 = Marmoreal. 2 = Waves. 3 = Amorphous. 4 = Color fringes.

The inadequate lipid layer in lens wearers is expected to contribute to both an increase in evaporation and to CLIDE. Pinching the lower eyelid margins with the fingers can squeeze more lipid out of the meibomian glands. After a few blinks this extra lipid is spread over the ocular surface increasing the overall thickness of the lipid layer (Craig *et al.*, 1995a). Simple manipulation of the lids can help in mild cases of dry eye. Synthetics and other pollutants in the air can react with the lipid layer, breaking it down leading to dry eye symptoms. Patients with dry-eye symptoms related to the work place may have an inadequate lipid layer (Franck, 1991; Franck & Palmvang, 1993). Before using any technique to assess the lipid layer in your patients, it is essential to obtain 'normal' values because they may be influenced by environmental factors in your own consulting room. A learning curve is associated with the subjective use of the Tearscope and there may be interoperator variations interpreting the interference patterns. Currently, the instrument is no longer marketed but this situation may change in the near future.

MEIBOMIOMETRY

The meibomian glands can be observed by appropriate lid eversion and retro-illumination using a suitable light source (Robin *et al.*, 1985). This is a useful way of recording the overall quality and gross morphology of the glands. The meibomian oil droplets seen at the orifices of the glands can be harvested using thin strips of grease-proof paper, and either the oils could be assayed, or the area of the meibomian impressions could be measured (Chew *et al.*, 1993). The area of the impression is an indication of lipid volume. Currently, the clinical value of meibomiometry in the busy primary care setting is questionable.

EVAPORIMETRY

Clearly, by definition, an evaporative dry eye has a greater than normal rate of evaporation from the ocular surface. Contact lenses disrupt the tear film and in turn increase tear evaporation and this may lead to CLIDE. Almost any drop instilled on the eye will increase evaporation rate and predispose the eye to dry eye symptoms either short or long term (Trees & Tomlinson, 1990). Many devices have been developed to measure tear evaporation (see for example Mathers *et al.*, 1993) still, most tear evaporimetry systems are cumbersome laboratory techniques based on the technology adapted for measuring evaporation from skin.

LACTOPLATE TEST

The lysozyme and lactoferrin are the dominant proteins secreted by the lacrimal glands. These proteins protect the ocular surface by virtue of their antibacterial properties. In lacrimal gland dysfunction the concentration of tear proteins is reduced. The Lactoplate™ test (Eagle Vision, USA) is a simple test for lactoferrin content. A small tear sample is taken from the lower fornix and placed on an immunodiffusive reactive plate. The sample diffuses outwards and forms a ring, in a manner akin to chromatography. The ring size is correlated with lactoferrin concentration. This test is popular in some countries but not available in UK. The test time is 3 days and only measures one property of the tears. However, as a secondary procedure it can be used when the clinician is convinced the patient has a dry eye but is unsure of the fundamental cause.

REFRACTOMETRY

The refractive index of a mixture depends on the refractive indices of the constituents of the mixture and their relative concentrations. The refractive index of pure proteins is approximately 1.55 and the refractive index of water is 1.333. In theory, the higher the protein concentration in tears, the higher the resulting refractive index. Stegman and Miller (1975) showed that, in experimental allergic conjunctivitis, tear protein levels are increased and this raised the tear refractive index. Furthermore, the refractive index of tears harvested from the lower tear meniscus from normal subjects has a direct relationship with tear lactoferrin concentration (Craig *et al.*, 1995b). Refractometry could prove to be a rapid objective indicator of lacrimal function by indicating protein concentration. A lowered tear refractive index has been reported in dry eyes (Golding & Brennan, 1991). Lactoferrin concentration in normal tear samples averages at 1.64 (S.D. ± 0.47) mg/ml (Craig *et al.*, 1995b) and by extrapolation it is estimated tear refractive index reduces by 0.00095 units for a 1 mg/ml fall in lactoferrin concentration (Patel *et al.*, 2000). For a refractometer to gain popularity in the clinical detection of dry eye, the reliability and repeatability should be less than 0.0001 units, the device should be objective and economically viable.

TEAR FERNING

When a tear sample is placed on a glass plate and allowed to dry out, the solid content of the sample precipitates forming an arborizing pattern (Kogbe *et al.*, 1991; Pennsyl & Dillehay, 1998). On a qualitative basis, these patterns can be graded and it appears, dry eyes have tear ferning patterns different from normals because of a reduced tear protein content. Monitoring tear ferning patterns could be useful in assessing the effects of treatment on dry eyes. Mathematical tools such as fractal analysis could be used to analyze the ferning pattern more precisely and as such may be developed into simplified clinical techniques allowing the clinician to objectively gauge the effect of tailored dry eye therapy in specific cases.

OSMOLALITY

Tear fluid consists of several constituents present in balanced harmony. The inorganic components such as sodium chloride, influence the osmotic pressure of the tear fluid and the concentration of these inorganic components is termed osmolality. Osmolality can be determined by measuring the freezing point of minute (e.g 0.3 μl) tear samples using a nanoliter osmometer. When lacrimal function is reduced the osmolality of tear samples taken from the tear menisci increases from a normal level of <312 mOsm/kg to >320 mOsm/kg (Craig, 1995). Many believe this technique should be the 'gold standard' for detecting the dry eye (Farris, 1994). Currently, osmometry is a laboratory procedure which, with suitable refinement, could be developed into a simple clinical test for assessing lacrimal function.

REFERENCES

Chew C.K.S., Jansweijer C., Tiffany J.M. *et al.* (1993). An instrument for quantifying meibomian lipid on the lid margin: The meibometer. *Curr Eye Res*, **12**: 247–254.

Craig J.P. (1995). Tear physiology in the normal and dry eye. PhD thesis, Glasgow Caledonian University, p 90.

Craig J.P. and Tomlinson A. (1997). Importance of the lipid layer in tear film stability and evaporation. *Optom Vis Sci*, **74**: 8–13.

Craig J.P., Blades K.J. and Patel S. (1995a). Tear lipid layer structure and stability following expression of the meibomian glands. *Ophthal Physiol Opt*, **15**: 569–574.

Craig J.P., Simmons P.A., Patel S. and Tomlinson A. (1995b). Refractive index and osmolality of human tears. *Optom Vis Sci*, **72**: 718–724.

Doane M.G. (1989). An instrument for in vivo tear film interferometry. *Optom Vis Sci*, **66**: 383–388.

Farris R.L. (1994). Tear osmolarity: A new gold standard. In: *The Preocular Tear Film in Health, Disease and Contact Lens Wear* (Holly F.J., ed.). Lubbock, Dry Eye, pp 495–503.

Franck C. (1991). Fatty layer of the precorneal film in the 'office eye syndrome'. *Acta Ophthalmol*, **69**: 737–743.

Franck C. and Palmvang I.B. (1993). Break-up time and lissamine green epithelial damage in 'office eye syndrome'. 6 month and one year follow-up. *Acta Ophthalmol*, **71**: 62–64s.

Golding T.R. and Brennan N.A. (1991). Tear refractive index in dry and normal eyes. *Clin Exp Optom*, **74**(suppl): 212.

Guillon J.P. and Guillon M. (1993). Tear film examination of the contact lens patient. *Optician*, **206**: 21–29.

King-Smith P.E., Fink B.A. and Fogt N. (1999). Three interferometric methods for measuring the thickness of layers of the tear film. *Optom Vis Sci*, **76**: 19–32.

Kogbe O., Liotet S. and Tiffany J.M. (1991). Factors responsible for tear ferning. *Cornea*, **10**: 433–444.

Mathers W.D., Binarao G. and Petroll M. (1993). Ocular evaporation and the dry eye: A new device. *Cornea*, **12**: 335–340.

Patel S., Boyd K.E. and Burns J. (2000). Age, stability of the precorneal tear film and the refractive index of tears. *Contact Lens Anterior Eye*, **23**: 44–47.

Patel S., Pérez-Santonja J.J., Alió J.L. and Murphy P.J. (2001). Corneal sensitivity and some properties of the tear film after LASIK. *J Refractive Surgery*, **17**: 17–24.

Pennsyl C.D. and Dillehay S.M. (1998). The repeatability of tear mucus ferning grading. *Optom Vis Sci*, **75**: 600–604.

Robin J.B., Jester J.V., Nobe J. *et al.* (1985). In vivo transillumination biomicroscopy and photography of meibomian gland dysfunction. *Ophthalmology*, **92**: 1423–1426.

Stegman R. and Miller D.A. (1975). A human model of allergic conjunctivitis. *Arch Ophthalmol*, **93**: 1354–1358.

Trees G.R. and Tomlinson A. (1990). Effect of artificial tear solutions and saline on tear film evaporation. *Optom Vis Sci*, **67**: 886–890.

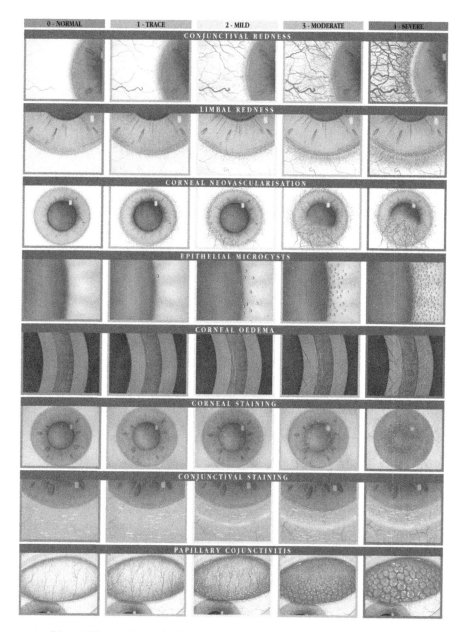

Plate 1 Efron grading scales. Rows 1 and 2 can be used to assess conjunctival health.

7 Ocular Surface Health

By the end of this chapter you will understand:

■ Why it is important to assess the health of the ocular surface;

■ How to assess the ocular surface.

When concerned with dry eye problems it is tempting to restrict discussion to only the tears (quantity and quality) or symptoms of dryness and discomfort. However, it must be remembered that the tears and the underlying ocular surface are completely interdependent. Although tissues such as the conjunctival epithelia are dependent on the tears, they are also responsible for aspects of tear film production and formation, so, a finely balanced mutual dependency exists. As a consequence, the corneal and conjunctival surfaces must be assessed when screening for dry eye, to complete the clinical picture. Likewise, the eyelids should not be forgotten. Examination of the eyelids can demonstrate causes of some dry eye problems. For example, lid deformations such as the one shown in Figure 7.1, can lead to incomplete spreading of the tears. Similarly, blocked meibomian glands (Figure 7.2), causing tear lipid deficiency are easily seen on examination.

HYPEREMIA ASSESSMENT

Conjunctival hyperemia (dilation of the episcleral vasculature) can be viewed as a barometer of ocular tissue response to provocative factors. Increased conjunctival hyperemia can be seen in response

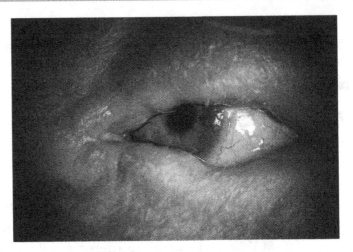

Figure 7.1 Congenital lid deformation. Poor lid configuration can lead to abnormal blinking, poor tear film and gross irritation.

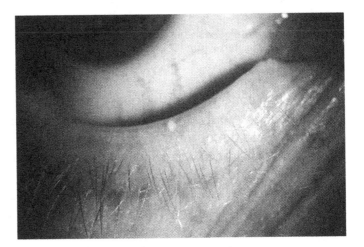

Figure 7.2 Blocked meibomian gland.

to prolonged toxic or physiological insult; lens surface deposits; contact lens degradation and episodes of infection. Assessment of conjunctival hyperemia is non-invasive, simple to perform, and offers a valuable insight into the general health of the anterior surface of the eye. Photographic scales have been developed to increase accuracy and repeatability of conjunctival hyperemia assessment.

Example hyperemia scale

There are several hyperemia scales to choose from, ranging from the widely available commercial scales (e.g. Efron Scale available from Hydron™ or the CCLRU scale available from Vistakon™) to

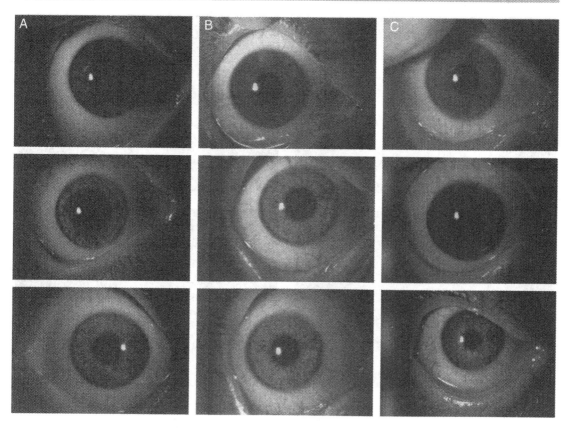

Figure 7.3 (A,B,C) GCU 9 point scale of conjunctival hyperemia. From none (0) to 9 (gross).

the proprietary (e.g. the GCU 9 Point scale of Hyperemia). These scales are reproduced in Plate 1 and in Figures 7.3 and 7.4.

The use of a standard, uniform light source, such as Burton lamp illumination or the use of a slit lamp at lowest magnification, with agreed assessment criteria may be advantageous when using a pictorial scale of this nature (McMonnies & Chapman-Davies, 1987).

It is a good idea to keep a copy of the same scale in each consulting room of a contact lens practice, and to routinely record hyperemia. Any marked changes noted from one patient visit to the next may warrant further investigation. These scales are subjective. The numerical value attached to a particular level of hyperemia is relative to the other categories of hyperemia noted in that scale. The values are relative, they are not absolute, and the scales are not interchangeable. It is good clinical practice to select a scale with which you feel confident and which represents the range normally presented by your patients. You should include one scale in your practice and stick to it! Having too many scales will inevitably lead to confusion and a mix up some time in the future.

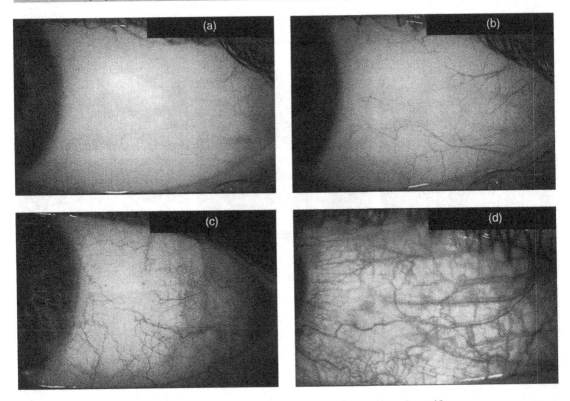

Figure 7.4 CCLRU scale of hyperemia. (a) Very slight (b) slight (c) moderate (d) severe.

OCULAR SURFACE STAINING

The extent of ocular surface damage can be easily assessed by instilling a small amount of Rose Bengal or fluorescein onto the ocular surface. It is usually the area within the lid aperture that is most likely to stain in dry eye stain (from scattered spots to large areas).

Fluorescein sodium (1% or 2%) stains areas of epithelial cell loss when instilled into the lower conjunctival sac. Rose Bengal (1%) stains dead epithelial cells and mucus. Corneal and conjunctival staining can be viewed by slit lamp, using a green filter. It is best to introduce only a very small amount of Rose Bengal onto the eye, because it irritates. Lissamine Green has been proposed as a less irritating alternative to Rose Bengal.

Van Bijsterveld's scoring system (1969) can be used to quantify the level of staining observed (with scores ranging from 0 to 9). This is shown in Figure 7.5 where the visible eye is divided into three zones, formed by imaginary vertical lines at either side of the limbus. Each zone is given a score depending upon the degree of

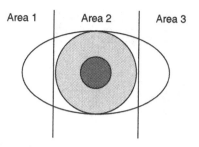

Figure 7.5 Zoning the ocular surface.

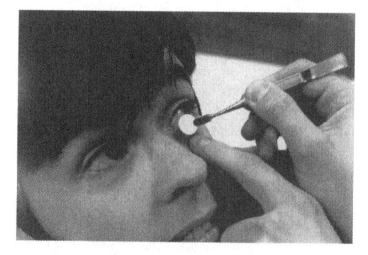

Figure 7.6 Conjunctival impression cytology – taking the impression. The millipore paper is gently pressed on the conjunctiva for a few seconds then removed.

staining contained, from 0 for no staining, through 1 for mild staining and 2 for moderate staining, to 3 for severe staining. A total score is calculated by adding the scores for the three zones of the ocular surface.

CONJUNCTIVA CELLULAR STATUS ASSESSMENT

Conjunctival impression cytology (CIC) is a minimally invasive technique allowing for the investigation of conjunctival changes, at the cellular level (Egbert *et al.*, 1977; Tseng, 1985; Nelson, 1988; Knop & Brewitt, 1992) (Figures 7.6–7.8). This technique involves pressing a piece of material, cellulose-acetate filters being a commonly used commercially available example, onto the bulbar or tarsal conjunctiva. The action of application and removal of the filter results in a fine sheet of superficial conjunctival epithelial tissue

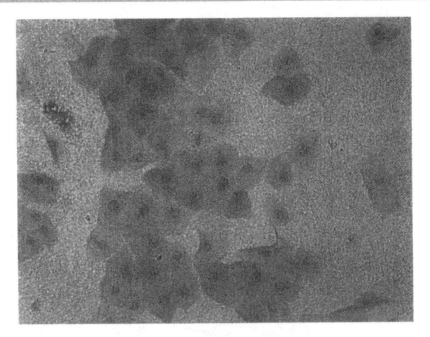

Figure 7.7 Conjunctival impression cytology from a dry eye. The low density of cells is common in dry eyes.

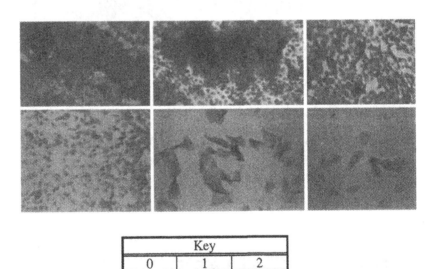

Key		
0	1	2
3	4	5

Figure 7.8 Tseng's squamous metaplasia scale. The extent of metaplasia can be graded qualitatively from 0 to 5.

remaining adhered to the filter. The adhered tissue can then be fixed and stained, and the visualized cells observed directly (light microscopy). It has been suggested that CIC may be useful in predicting success or failure in contact lens wear (Hirji & Larke, 1981). To date, this has not been proven however, using CIC the conjunctival goblet cell count in dry eye is definitely reduced (see for example, Sullivan *et al.*, 1973; Nelson & Wright, 1986).

The sensation felt when the filter is applied is similar to that experienced on the first fitting of a contact lens (due to the presence of a foreign body and the inability to blink), and slight irritation is felt as the filter is removed. Topical anesthetic can be used to minimize discomfort. The key to good subject tolerance of this technique lies in a confident and rapid cell collection following a full explanation of the technique.

Goblet cell population density can be assessed by impression cytology if the goblet cell contents are stained specifically, e.g. using periodic acid schiff. A low goblet cell population density is thought to indicate inability to produce a sufficient mucus phase of the tear film, as the major proportion of this layer is produced by the goblet cells. However, no demonstration of a direct relationship between goblet cell numbers and the conjunctiva's ability to produce ocular mucus has been made. By inference, however, a cause–effect relationship is assumed.

The extent of conjunctival squamous metaplasia is another index of conjunctival health, which can be assessed following CIC sample collection. This parameter indicates the 'health' and integrity of the conjunctiva as a mucous membrane: many dry eye states are accompanied with a morphological shift towards keratinization of the conjunctival epithelium. While conjunctival keratinization may be a defensive measure, protecting against conjunctival desiccation in the absence of sufficient tear volume or quality, this morphological alteration is almost definitely detrimental to the conjunctiva in terms of its ability to function correctly for the maintenance of the tear film's functional and physical integrity. Increased squamous metaplasia is normally associated with a decrease in conjunctival goblet cell density (see Figure 7.8). Using CIC conjunctival cell count tends to reduce in both rigid and soft lens wearers as demonstrated in Figure 7.9. Even in daily disposable soft lens wear, conjunctival cell count is below normal (Connors *et al.*, 1997), predisposing wearers to dry eye. Dry eye can also manifest itself in marked alterations in the appearance of conjunctival cells' nuclei, leading to the appearance of 'snake like chromatin'.

While it is tempting to propose impression cytology as a clinical test for dry eye, this technique is still very much a laboratory technique. While it is easy and quick to collect the 'impression' material, staining and assessing the sample is too time consuming and involved for routine clinical practice. However, if diagnostic guidelines regarding assessment of impressions can be established, and a simplified

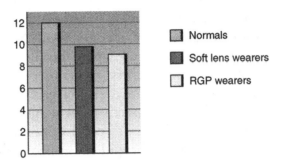

Figure 7.9 Conjunctival goblet cell count in normal and symptom free veteran daily contact lens wearers. Normals, $n = 9$, average age 27.1 years (s.d. = ±6.5 years). Soft lens (SL) wearers, $n = 8$, average age 32.3 years (s.d. = ±10.2 years), wearing HEMA lenses on daily basis for an average of 8.5 years (s.d. = ±4.8 years). Rigid lens (RGP) wearers, $n = 7$, average age 31.7 years (s.d. = ±9.6 years), wearing low DK lenses on daily basis for average of 10.6 years (s.d. = ±9.1 years). Goblet cell count noted as % of total lens count per CIC sample. Samples taken from superior bulbar conjunctiva. Between normals and RGP subjects difference is significant ($p = 0.045$). Between normals and SL subjects, $p = 0.167$ (Blades, Murphy and Patel, 1994).

staining protocol can be accepted, then conjunctival impression cytology could find its way into clinical practice in the future.

SUMMARY

Because the ocular surface and tear film are intrinsically related, ocular surface assessment must not be forgotten. Currently accepted techniques of conjunctival hyperemia assessment and ocular surface staining assessment are quick and easy. In the future, clinicians could routinely assess ocular surface changes at the cellular level, if impression cytology can be adapted for clinical utility.

REFERENCES

Blades K., Murphy P.J. and Patel S. (1994). Status of conjunctival goblet cells in contact lens wearers. *Optom and Vis Sci*, 71s(12) (suppl): 95.

Connors C.G., Campbell J.B. and Steel S.A. (1997). The effects of disposable wear contact lenses on goblet cell count. *CLAOJ*, 23: 37–39.

Egbert P.R., Lauber S. and Maurice D.M. (1977). A simple conjunctival biopsy. *Am J Ophthalmol*, 84: 798–801.

Hirji N.K. and Larke J.R. (1981). Conjunctival impression cytology in contact lens practice. *J Brit Cont Lens Assoc*, 4: 159–161.

Knop E. and Brewitt H. (1992). Induction of conjunctival epithelial alterations by contact lens wearing. A prospective study. *Ger J Ophthalmol*, 1: 125–134.

McMonnies C.W. and Chapman-Davies A. (1987). Assessment of conjunctival hyperemia in contact lens wearers: Parts I & II. *Am J Optom Physiol Opt*, 64: 246–255.

Nelson J.D. (1988). Impression cytology. *Cornea*, 7: 71–81.

Nelson J.D. and Wright J.C. (1986). Impression cytology of the ocular surface in keratoconjunctivitis sicca. In: *The Preocular Tear Film in Health, Disease and Contact Lens Wear* (Holly F.J., ed.). Dry Eye Inst, Lubbock, Tx, pp 140–156.

Sullivan W.R., McCulley J.P. and Dohlman C.H. (1973). Return of goblet cells after vitamin A therapy in xerosis of the conjunctiva. *Am J Ophthalmol*, 75: 720–725.

Tseng S.C. (1985). Staging a conjunctival squamous metaplasia by impression cytology. *Ophthalmology*, 92: 728–733.

Van Bijisterveld O.P. (1969). Diagnostic tests in the sicca syndrome. *Arch Ophthalmol*, 82: 10–14.

8 Treatment of Dry Eye

By the end of this chapter you will understand:

■ The key features in the development of modern methods for combating dry eye problems;

■ The limitations of the commonly used techniques;

■ How to develop a dry eye treatment strategy for your patient.

The various treatments for dry eye are aimed at substituting, preserving or stimulating production of tears. This chapter will focus on treating dry eye in primary care with a short reference on more advanced pharmacological treatments normally meted out on severe dry eyes within the secondary care sector.

The care of the dry eye is directly associated with the exact cause of the problem. Thus, it is imperative that you, the clinician, investigate and arrive at some answers to account for your patient's symptoms. Armed with this knowledge, you can combat the patient's symptoms more effectively and this will raise the patient's confidence in you. On many occasions the symptoms are due to poor hygiene. Ocular washouts, especially after sleep, and lid scrubs can be all the patient needs. The most popular dry eye treatments include artificial tear drops and supplements.

ARTIFICIAL TEARS

There are several artificial tear drop (ATD) formulations designed to compensate for either lacrimal or mucous insufficiency. Most ATDs act as tear substitutes. Internation variations in legislation has led to the situation whereby, in some countries some drops are prescription only and in others they can be sold over the counter. In this chapter we will not list the various artificial tear drops available in, say, the UK simply because the list would soon become out of date as new products are introduced and others are withdrawn at a rapid rate compared with other therapeutic agents. Most drops contain preservatives and in many cases the drops exacerbate symptoms because of patient hypersensitivity to the preservatives. Single-dose preservative-free drops appear as a more expensive option, however this is not always the case. Most preserved drops should be discarded 28 days after opening. If the dry eye problem is occasional say on 2 or 3 times per week, then a 20 or 30 dose pack would last a lot longer and offer a much better cost-effective choice to the patient. The value of artificial tears can be assessed very rapidly using one or more of the simple tests described in Chapters 2, 3–6 for investigating the dry eye. Figures 8.1–8.3 show the effects of a preservative-free tear drop (Vislube™ by Chemidica) on tear stability, meniscus height and lipid layer. Clearly the drop is improving the status of the preocular tear film. When a single drop is instilled onto the ocular surface the bulk of its volume rapidly drains away via the naso-lacrimal duct. In effect only a minute amount of the initial drop is of real value in terms of ocular surface wetting and lubrication. When using a single dose sachet, ask the patient to tilt the head back, instil a drop on one eye, wait a few moments, and then instil the other eye. There will still be fluid remaining in the sachet, wait a few moments more and repeat. This is a useful way of making maximum use of the drops.

With most ATDs the increase in tear stability peaks approximately 15 minutes after instillation. Thereafter, the tear stability reduces and reaches baseline about 90 minutes later. In the case of pre-soft lens tear stability some in-eye wetting drops improve stability but the effect lasts no more than 5 minutes (Golding *et al.*, 1990). Many investigations claim that persistent use of drops can produce a longer-lasting improved baseline in tear stability. This could be mediated by either:

1. a healing effect or;
2. return of the epithelial surface to a more natural state or;
3. gradual repopulation of active conjunctival goblet cells.

On instillation, ATDs can momentarily blur the patient's vision. If the drop has a refractive index radically different from the refractive index of natural tears and the drop mixes poorly with the tears, the instilled drop will scatter light in the direction towards the retina. In turn this affects the quality of the retinal image and

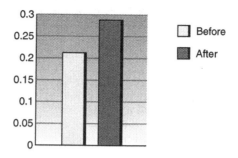

Figure 8.1 TMH (mm) before and after using Vislube™ ($n = 15$, $t = 2.21$, $p = 0.035$, S.D. $= \pm0.09$ before and ±0.098 after).

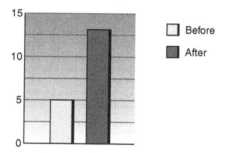

Figure 8.2 TTT (seconds) before and after Vislube™ ($n = 40$, $W = 1140.5$, $p = 0.00001$).

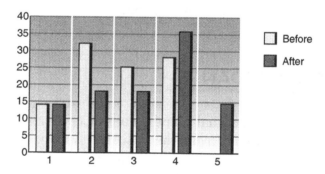

Figure 8.3 Lipid layer category before and after Vislube™ ($n = 40$, $W = 134.5$, $p > 0.05$). 1 = no lipid, 2 = marmoreal, 3 = waves, 4 = amorphous, 5 = color fringes.

hence vision. Some patients find this disturbing at critical viewing times (e.g. driving, VDT use). Highly viscous drops and ointment are the worse offenders. The refractive index values of some popular ATDs are listed in Table 8.1. Clearly, some are more likely to affect vision than others. In common with most other eye drops, artificial tears are buffered to maintain a pH close to the pH of natural tears. Depending on the concentration of the instilled drop the eye can tolerate comfortably a pH range from 6.6. to 7.8 (Milder, 1975; Carney & Fullard, 1979). Thus, the pH of artificial tears

Table 8.1 Refractive index and pH of some artificial tears

Drop	Refractive index	pH
Viva-Drops	1.3354	6.7
Hypromellose	1.3347	8.2
SNO-Tears	1.3357	5.3
Tears naturelle	1.3339	6.5
Isopto-Plain	1.3351	7.4
Hypo-tears (UK)	1.3391	5.9
Celluvisc	1.3351	6.4
Refresh	1.3342	6.2
Visco-Tears	1.3376	7.1
Clerz	1.3352	7.4
Genteal	1.3332	6.7
Ocucoat	1.3346	7.2
Hypotears (USA)	1.3393	5.5
Optifree rewetting drops	1.3337	6.9

1. Refractive index measured using S-10 refractometer (Atago, Japan).
2. pH measured using pH Meter model 10 (Corning-Eel Scientific Instruments).
3. All samples were fresh, previously unused and measured at room temperature (25°C).

should fall within these limits. Table 8.1 lists the measured pH of various ATDs, all measurements were taken under masked randomized conditions. In theory some ATDs will be more acceptable in terms of comfort compared with others.

ORAL ANTIOXIDANTS

The lacrimal glands, conjunctivae and meibomian glands obtain nutrients from the vascular system. A number of quintessential anti-oxidants are prominent in the biochemical processes leading to the manufacture and secretion of the essential tear constituents. Vitamins A, C, E, zinc, selenium and molybdenum together with other key nutrients prominently feature in tear metabolism. It has been shown, within a 'normal, healthy, symptom-free' population group, that the blood plasma levels of essential antioxidants such as vitamin C can be so low that they reach near pathological levels (Johnston & Thompson, 1998). Other than injecting nutrients directly into the blood stream we could reach these tissues via the digestive tract. Within 'a normal, allegedly healthy, symptom-free' population group, either vitamin C (1000 mg/day), vitamin A (2250 μg/day) or an anti-oxidant mixture (1 tablet/day

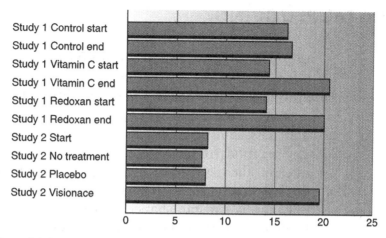

Figure 8.4 Changes in tear stability with systemic antioxidants. **Study 1**: (Patel et al., 1993a). 60 asymptomatic student subjects/(30F, 30M) average age 20 years. Single masked randomized design, subjects divided into equal groups, one treated with vitamin C, one with Redoxan™ (LaRoche) one with no treatment (control). Treatment for 10 days. Each vitamin C tablet contained 1000 mg. **Study 2**: (Blades et al., 2001). 40 marginal dry eye subjects (30F, 10M) average age 53 years ($\pm$15.3). Masked randomized trial with cross-over design. 1 month of active treatment, 1 month of placebo, 1 month with no treatment. Active treatment consisted of 2 tablets of VisionACE™ (Vitabiotics Ltd) daily. Content of each Redoxan™ tablet: Vitamins A (1500 μg), B1 (15 μg), B2 (5 μg), B6 (11.6 μg), B12 (5 μg), C (150 μg), D (10 μg), E (50 μg), Calcium (1.25 μg), Iron (1.25 μg), Magnesium (5 μg), Copper (0.5 μg), Zinc (0.5 μg), Molybdenum (0.1 μg), Manganese (0.5 μg), Niacin (50 μg), Pantothenic acid (11.6 μg), Biotin (250 μg), Folic acid (300 μg), Phosphate (45 μg). Content of each VisionACE™ tablet: β-Carotene (6 mg), Vitamins E (120 mg), C (300 mg), B6 (30 mg), D (5 μg), B1 (15 mg), B2 (10 mg), B12 (9 μg), K (200 μg), Folic acid (500 μg), Pantothenic acid (20 mg), Magnesium (100 mg), Zinc (15 mg), Iron (6 mg), Iodine (200 μg), Copper (2 mg), Manganese (4 mg), Selenium (200 μg), Chromium (100 μg), Cystine (40 mg), Methionine (40 mg), Bioflavinoids (30 mg).

of Redoxan™, La Roche) can substantially improve tear stability after 7–10 days of treatment (Patel et al., 1993a, 1993b). In a controlled study featuring placebo and cross-over design, oral ingestion of the antioxidant mixture VisionACE™ (Vitabiotics, UK) for 1 month substantially improved both tear stability and goblet cell count in symptomatic marginal dry eyes (Blades et al., 2001). The key features of these studies are shown in Figure 8.4.

Tear drops and ointments containing vitamin A (or its analogs) are available for direct application to the ocular surface. Vitamin A is fat soluble, therefore, it should be supplied in a suitable non-aqueous medium. Aqueous tear drops containing vitamin A have such a low vitamin A content that it is difficult to believe these preparations do any good other than act as a placebo. If these drops do improve ocular surface health then the cause is probably the lubricant vehicle not the vitamin A.

PUNCTAL PLUGGING

When the dry eye is due to insufficient aqueous production and other, less obtrusive, methods have been tried and found to be insufficient then, punctal plugging should be attempted. Aimed at preserving the tears, several plugs are available in various sizes, materials, construction, and they are often supplied with an intricate method for insertion. The Herrick plug is fabricated from flexible silicone rubber, it is peg-shaped and supplied with a thin flexible wire inserter. The Freeman plug is made from a harder polymer, is capstan-shaped and has an intricate assembly which facilitates insertion. Punctal plugs wider than the actual puncta are normally fitted to rest tight in the lacrimal canals. If the plug is too narrow it would simply pass down the canals by the massaging effects produced by the lid muscles by the constant blinking and natural eye movements.

To insert a plug, simply dilate the punctum using a Foster dilator. The sterile dilator is a tapered blunt pin. Passing it down the punctum and rotating with the hand and gently pushing from side to side will widen the punctum. Topical anesthesia and a drop of lubricant can be useful but this is not mandatory. The Freeman plug fitting assembly has a plug dilator incorporated in its design. The plug is pushed down the punctum and turned through 90 degrees past the apex of the L-shaped canal. When using the Freeman plug, the plug release assembly is pressed between the fingers, this frees the plug and the applicator assembly is gently withdrawn from the canal. For the Herrick plug, once it is inside the canal, the wire is gently rotated and pulled back. The fluted end of the Herrick plug in contact with the walls of the canal is held in place by friction as the wire is gently withdrawn.

Temporary collagen plugs should be used initially as a provocative test that allows the clinician to gauge the value of a more prolonged punctal therapy and allows the patient a chance to experience the benefits or otherwise. These are manufactured from porcine collagen and some patients may decline these plugs on religious or other grounds. The plug should be the same or one step wider than the punctum. The punctum is dilated as described, the prepacked sterile plug is gripped between the pincers of sterilized fine jeweller's forceps, the eyelid is pulled back to reveal a gaping punctum and the plug is inserted into the punctum. Once the plug touches the lid margin, it soaks up tears and expands. A swelling plug will become difficult to insert, hence it is advised to get the plug in as a 'hole-in-one'. Once inserted, the plug should be gently pushed down into the canal until it is no longer visible to the clinician. The swelling of the inserted plug keeps it in place and prevents extrusion.

Tear stability and meniscus height should be measured prior to punctal plugging. The collagen plug will dissolve within a week or so, it is useful to check the patient within 48 hours. Both tear stability and meniscus height should be re-evaluated. Patients very quickly realize whether the plug is doing any good. If the patient complains of epiphora then rest assured the plug will dissolve away in a few days. Ideally, if the plug is working, patient symptoms and tear characteristics will initially improve and fall back towards baseline as the plug gradually dissolves.

The collagen plugs are also useful for frequent flyers and patients susceptible to the dry conditions in air-conditioned hotels. Many patients have annoying dry eye symptoms when traveling in airplanes. In these cases, fitting collagen plugs before a long-haul flight can be beneficial. Changes in selected tear properties in a particular case of an 80-year-old female patient are shown in Figures 8.5 and 8.6.

Some clinicians prefer occluding all four puncta. However, in the author's opinion, plugging the lower puncta is sufficient in most cases because the bulk of tears drains away to the naso-lacrimal duct via this route. Occasionally, plugs can end up ejected from the canaliculi. After 6–14 months, in about 1% of cases the plug may pass out the punctum (Fayat *et al.*, 2001). It could be lost by passing into the nasal cavity. In extreme cases, the puncta may be sealed with cautery or cyanoacrylate adhesives.

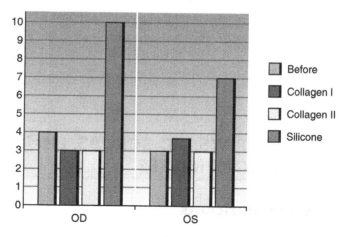

Figure 8.5 Case history. Change in TTT in an 80-year-old female with severe dry eyes treated with collagen and Herrick™ punctal plugs. TTT before and after collagen and silicone plugs. Start, 2 days and 1 week with collagen. Then, 1 week with silicone.

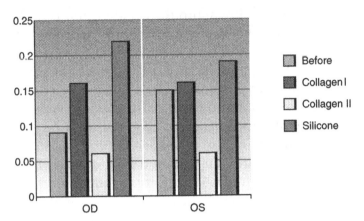

Figure 8.6 Case history. Change in TMH in an 80-year-old female with severe dry eyes treated with collagen and Herrick™ punctal plugs. TTT before and after collagen and silicone plugs. Start, 2 days and 1 week with collagen. Then, 1 week with silicone.

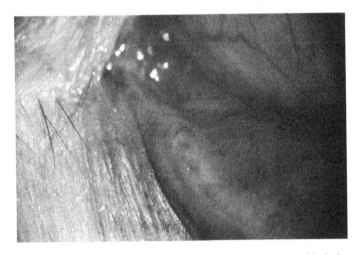

Figure 8.7 Case of two puncta at a lower eyelid. Both puncta are blocked.

A patient may present with two lower puncta as shown in Figure 8.7. This is rare however; both canaliculae should be investigated in case one is vestigial.

OINTMENTS, SPRAYS, LID SCRUBS, LID THERAPY, SIDESHIELDS, COMPRESSES

Ointments and lubricants

Ointments and lubricants either prevent ocular surface friction damage, retain fluid or maintain surface hydration. If the patient tends to sleep with the eyes partially open, an ointment at bedtime is called for. Similarly, ointments are useful in superficial ocular surface damage.

Lid scrubs

Lid scrubs are useful for cleaning the lid margin at the junction between the skin and palpebral conjunctiva, unblocking meibomian gland openings, removing environmental debris (pollution), make-up, dry skin, denatured skin and mucosal secretions. Scrubs are useful in cases of mild blepharitis or meibomitis. Also, lid massaging forces fresh meibomian secretions to pass through the duct openings.

Sprays

Liposomal sprays are claimed, by the manufacturers, to enhance the skin and mucous membranes. The spray is made up microvesicles consisting of an inner aqueous phase and an outer phospholipid bi-layer floating in an aqueous outer phase. Their use produces a refreshing sensation, however the manufacturer's claims have yet to be substantiated by proper clinical trials.

Lid therapy

Lid therapy is suitable when the dry eye symptoms are of environmental origin. Gently pinching the lower or upper lid margin will sqeeze meibomian oils out onto the ocular surface. After a few blinks, the extra lipid is spread over the precorneal tear film, thickening the lipid layer (Craig *et al.*, 1995) and this should in turn reduce the evaporation of tears from the ocular surface. In cases where the meibomian secretions are insufficiently soft and viscous, hot compresses or hot spoon presses can soften the secretions by raising the temperature. This eases the passage of the meibomian oils to the ocular surface.

Surface protection

In extreme cases, patients may find goggles helpful in maintaining high levels of humidity around the eyes. Disposable clear, semi-rigid goggles designed to fit over one eye (e.g. 'the dry eye comforter' by Solan™ Ophthalmic Products, Jacksonville FL, USA) are useful during sleep and in the rare cases of monocular dry eye. Sometimes, flexible side shields can be fitted to the patient's spectacles.

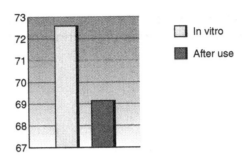

Figure 8.8 Change in water content of protective bandage hydrogel contact lenses.
(1) Water content inferred by measuring lens refractive index using a refractometer and converting the values to percentage water content using a pre-calibrated scale.
(2) 11 unused lenses (in vitro), 26 worn lenses (worn on an extended wear basis for less than 3 months). Measurements taken at room temperature (20–23°C). Difference in mean water content significant ($p < 0.05$).
(3) PSL 72%™ (polyvinyl pyrolidone) lenses supplied by Prospect Contact Lenses, UK.

Condensation can build up behind lenses, reducing vision and this may prove intolerable.

Bandage lenses

When the dry eye is severe leading to painful ocular surface damage and recurrent surface erosion, bandage lenses worn on an extended-wear basis could be considered. Bandage lenses protect the ocular surface in cases where either blinking causes more harm to the corneal epithelium, or the corneal epithelium is weakly fixed to the basement membrane. In keeping with other hydrogel lenses, high water content bandage lenses dehydrate when worn. A lipid layer is either non-existent or very thin over a soft lens (see Chapter 6, Figure 6.5) thus, during use, water evaporates from the bandage lens surface. This would lead to a shift in hydrostatic pressure along the thickness of the bandage and this in turn may draw water from the tears and into the bandage lens. Under steady-state conditions there is a continuous flow of water from the tears into the lens and out through the lens surface into the surrounding air. In some patients this would exasperate an already difficult situation. If all else fails, the patient could be referred for tarsorraphy. The typical changes occurring in the water content of bandage lenses are shown in Figure 8.8.

WATERY EYE

A watery eye can be just as troublesome as a dry eye. The drainage may be impeded because of narrowed or completely closed puncta.

The puncta tend to narrow with advancing years but this does not, in itself, mean the patient will develop a watery eye. In some cases, the puncta gradually become closed and vascularized but the tear meniscus height may remain within normal limits. In such cases, the closing of the puncta is to the patient's advantage – possibly a compensatory mechanism working to maintain equilibrium in cases where tear evaporation rate is elevated and tear production rate is depressed.

Punctal dilation and/or naso-lacrimal drainage should be attempted when the watery eye is a major source of discomfort and all other likely causes have been ruled out. The tissue immediately around the punctum is anesthetized with one drop of 0.4% benoxinate hydrochloride (or equivalent in, say, Minims form). A Foster punctum finder/dilator is cleaned and sterilized and inserted into the punctum, and rotated to widen the punctal aperture. This step is the same as the first step prior to inserting a punctal plug. The dilator is turned through 90 degrees towards the nose and passed along the lacrimal canal for about 5–10 mm. Rotate the dilator for a few seconds to stretch and widen the canal. The dilator is then withdrawn. With the punctum now opened up, a disposable syringe filled with 0.9% saline is fitted with a lacrimal cannula. With the patient's head tilted back, the cannula is inserted down into the lower punctum and passed into the canal in the same way as the dilator. The syringe is depressed to gently express saline into the canal. Some force may be required if the blockage is severe. After a little practice you will soon realize how much pressure you have to apply. Once the blockage is removed, the saline will pass into the nasal cavity, however when the head is tilted back gravity will cause the saline to dribble to the back of the throat and the patient will feel and taste the saline. This is a good practical indicator that saline has got through the drainage system. The procedure is now repeated on the other eye. Figure 8.9 shows a cannula in place in the lower punctum during a drainage procedure. The same punctum is shown immediately after the procedure in Figure 8.10. Clearly, the punctum is wide and definitely open however, in the author's opinion, a single attempt at lacrimal drainage is insufficient. The patient should return for a repeat procedure a week later. The tear meniscus height, size and shape of the punctum should be measured before and after each drainage session. These data are useful for gauging the value of your procedures. Some patients require three visits for practical restoration of drainage and sufficient relief of symptoms. The Jones' test could be used to check for patency of the drainage system. The authors prefer checking symptoms, TMH

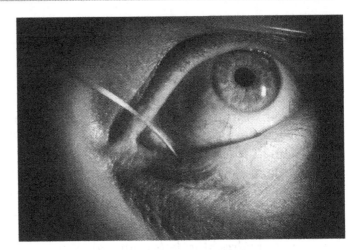

Figure 8.9 Lacrimal drainage. Cannula inserted in lower punctum after dilation. Cannula is swung towards the temporal side before saline is released.

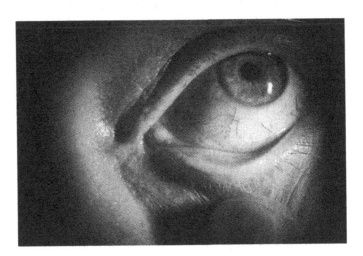

Figure 8.10 On removing the cannula. The punctum is now wide and open.

and dimensions of the puncta – these checks are quicker, less labor-intensive, less cumbersome, amenable to photo-documentation and more comfortable for the patient. The reduction in TMH values in three cases of watery eye after lacrimal procedures is shown in Figure 8.11, together with one case where the procedure was unsuccessful.

When drainage procedures fail flexible balloon catheters can be used to open up the drainage channel. The Lacricath™ (Corinthian Medical Ltd, Sutton-in-Ashfield, Notts, UK) is a catheter fitted with a small miniature balloon. The probe is passed into the naso-lacrimal duct and the balloon can be inflated up to 3 mm in diameter

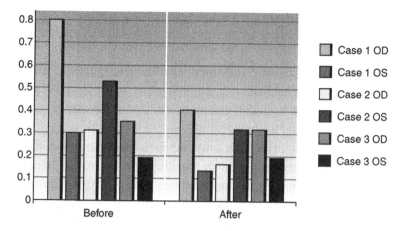

Figure 8.11 Case histories. TMH before and 1 week after punctal dilation and drainage procedure. Three cases, two successful and one unsuccessful [case 3].

when a pressure of 115 psi is applied. Patients with watery eye should be referred for more intensive ophthalmological intervention in the following situations.

i) When the blockage is hard and compact, the saline will be forced back and spout out onto the ocular surface. When the obstruction is persistent, an X-ray may be required to pinpoint the exact location and source of the blockage. More aggressive procedures such as incisional surgery and fitting a stent may be required to create a new passage for drainage. Laser-assisted surgery is becoming more popular and this may replace some of these invasive techniques.

ii) If the punctum is thickly vascularized and there is a likelihood of bleeding.

iii) Loss of tonus within the lower lid can lead to floppy eyelid and impaired tear retention and drainage. The patient should be referred to a surgeon specializing in oculo-plastics.

PHARMACOLOGICAL INTERVENTION

Ointments or solutions containing relatively high concentrations of vitamin A may be prescribed for direct application to the ocular surface in severe dry eyes. Some are prepared by hospital pharmacists, because preparatory brands are not widely available in the UK (e.g Vitamin a Dispersa from Dispersa containing 3.44 mg/g of retinyl acetate). In advanced dry eyes where the ocular surface is persistently irritated, cytokines are released leading to inflammation and neuronal impairment. Thus, in severe dry eyes we normally find:

i) chronic inflammation of the lacrimal glands, ocular surface and lids;
ii) a breakdown in the neuronal control of tear secretion.

Drugs that can combat inflammation and stimulate tear production by reversing or by-passing the neuronal breakdown have been used in these patients. For example, anti-inflammatory agents such as oral tetracyclines are useful for treating severe blepharitis particularly where there is corneal involvement (Frucht-Pery *et al.*, 1993) and topical cyclosporin A is useful because of its immunomodulating properties (Sall *et al.*, 2000; Stevenson *et al.*, 2000). Though widely used for other ophthalmic purposes, *Botulinum* toxin injected into the eyelids appears to decrease tear drainage and increase tear flow (Spiera *et al.*, 1997; Sahlin *et al.*, 2000) and may prove more popular in the future.

REFERENCES

Blades K.J., Patel S. and Aidoo K.E. (2001). Oral antioxidant therapy for marginal dry eye. *Eur J Clin Nutrition*, **55**: 589–597.

Carney L.G. and Fullard R.J. (1979). Ocular irritation and environmental pH. *Aust J Optom*, **62**: 335–336.

Craig J., Blades K.J. and Patel S. (1995). Tear lipid layer structure and stability following expression of the meibomian glands. *Opthal and Physiol Opt*, **15**: 569–574.

Fayat B., Assouline M., Hanush S. *et al.* (2001). Silicone punctal plug extrusion resulting from spontaneous dissection of canicular mucosa. *Ophthalmology*, **108**: 405–409.

Frucht-Pery J., Sagi E., Hemo I. and Ever-Hadani P. (1993). Efficacy of doxycycline and tetracycline in ocular rosacea. *Am J Ophthalmol*, **116**: 88–92.

Golding T.R., Efron N. and Brennan N.A. (1990). Soft lens lubricants and pre-lens tear lens tear stability. *Optom Vis Sci*, **67**: 461–465.

Johnston C.S. and Thompson L.L. (1998). Vitamin C status of an outpatient population. *J Am Coll Nutr*, **17**: 366–370.

Milder B. (1975). The lacrimal apparatus. In: *Adler's Physiology of the Eye* (Moses R.A., ed.). St. Louis, CV Mosby.

Patel S., Plaskow J. and Ferrier C. (1993a). The influence of vitamins and trace element supplements on the stability of the precorneal tear film. *Acta Ophthalmol*, **71**: 825–829.

Patel S., Asfar A.J. and Nabili S. (1993b). Effects of vitamin A on the stability of the precorneal tear film. *Optom Vis Sci* **70**(12 suppl): 64.

Sall K., Stevenson O.D., Mundorf T.K., Reis B.L. and the CsA Phase 3 Study Group. (2000). Two multicenter, randomized studies of the efficacy and safety of cyclosporin ophthalmic emulsion in moderate to severe dry eye disease. *Ophthalmology*, **107**: 631–639.

Sahlin S., Chen E., Kaugesaar T. *et al.* (2000). Effect of eyelid botulinum toxin injection on the lacrimal drainage. *Am J Ophthalmol*, **129**: 481–486.

Spiera H., Asbell P.A. and Simpson D.M. (1997). Botulinum toxin increases tearing in patients with Sjogren's syndrome: a preliminary report. *J Rheumatol*, **24**: 1842–1843.

Stevenson D., Tauber J. and Reis B.L. (2000). The Cyclosporin A Phase 2 study group: Efficacy and safety of cyclosporin A ophthalmic emulsion in the treatment of moderate-to-severe dry eye disease. A dose-ranging, randomized trial. *Ophthalmology*, **107**: 967–974.

Index

Note: Page numbers in *italics* refers to figures and tables.

Printed in the United States
By Bookmasters